Probl ...ook for Nurses

Dedication

To Helen and Tom for their support and patience.

Problem-Based Learning: A Handbook for Nurses

Kay Wilkie

and

Iain Burns

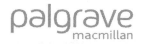
palgrave
macmillan

First published 2003 by
PALGRAVE MACMILLAN
Houndmills, Basingstoke, Hampshire RG21 6XS and
175 Fifth Avenue, New York, N.Y. 10010
Companies and representatives throughout the world

PALGRAVE MACMILLAN is the global academic imprint of the Palgrave Macmillan division of St. Martin's Press, LLC and of Palgrave Macmillan Ltd. Macmillan® is a registered trademark in the United States, United Kingdom and other countries. Palgrave is a registered trademark in the European Union and other countries.

ISBN 0–333–94577–8

This book is printed on paper suitable for recycling and made from fully managed and sustained forest sources.

A catalogue record for this book is available from the British Library.

10   9   8   7   6   5   4   3   2   1
12   11   10   09   08   07   06   05   04   03

Printed in Great Britain by J. W. Arrowsmith Ltd, Bristol.

Contents

List of Figures

Foreword

Problem solving lies at the heart of modern nursing. It is the professional nurse's ability to seek out the answers and provide the best possible care that separates the nurse from non-professional colleagues. And it is exactly these skills of enquiry that problem-based learning (PBL) will help students develop – skills that will be as much value in practice as they are in the classroom.

PBL is a relatively new educational approach – and already there are way too many definitions! But in essence I'm sure most would agree that PBL is more about students learning how to think about nursing and how to approach challenging situations, rather than providing all the answers. The other key component of PBL is that it is firmly grounded in reality – presenting students with real life scenarios that need to be approached from a social as well as a clinical perspective.

The emphasis on students learning how to learn, rather than passively receiving information in lectures, is challenging to both students and teachers – calling for a shift in emphasis from traditional teacher-student roles. Yet this shift is critical if we are to fulfil the demands of the modern NHS, which requires students to become more critical and active in their clinical decision-making.

This book offers a frank, jargon-busting and infinitely readable introduction to PBL. Since the authors look at PBL from both facilitator (staff) and student perspectives, their book can be used successfully by both groups. Its clear structure and succinct approach also allow readers to dip in and out, and easily pinpoint the information most relevant to their particular needs.

Through their own experiences of introducing PBL into a pre-registration nursing curriculum, the authors are well aware of the many different obstacles to implementation – practical, organisational and cultural. Thankfully they also have a good understanding of how these can be overcome, and offer invaluable information on the various approaches universities can take to issues such as staffing, timetabling, and evaluation.

Skilful facilitators are key to PBL. The authors rightly stress that most staff will need support to make the transition from lecturing to facilitating and their book offers a comprehensive starting point. It provides the basic framework and processes for establishing a programme; indicates the key issues to consider when introducing it into the curriculum; shows how PBL can be used creatively to encourage critical thinking; how to address negativity or unproductivity within the team; and ultimately how to evaluate how well the programme is working.

Students will also find the book a useful guide to PBL – enabling them to understand its underpinning philosophy, how to approach the learning process itself, and get the most out of it for the benefit of their own professional development and lifelong learning skills. Each chapter contains exercises which adopt the PBL approach, helping to further familiarise students with this method of learning. The book also provides practical tips on researching, from surfing the web to literature review.

Problem-based learning looks set to quickly gather momentum in nursing education over the next few years; I believe this is very good news for the future of modern healthcare. I commend this book to all involved in the education and training of nurses as a comprehensive and inspiring guide to PBL. I also recommend it highly to student nurses unfamiliar or new to PBL.

SALLY GLEN
Professor of Nursing Education and Dean,
St Bartholomew School of Nursing and Midwifery,
City University

Preface

This book is intended as a guide for those involved in developing, implementing and facilitating problem-based learning (PBL) in nursing curricula. It is designed to offer practical advice for both teachers and students engaged in PBL. It draws on our own experiences of introducing PBL into a pre-registration nursing curriculum within the higher education sector of United Kingdom during the period 1997–2001.

In introducing PBL as a development that moved from a traditional teacher-led, subject-based approach to nurse education to a problem-based, student-centred approach, we encountered many challenges. These included the need for academic staff to adopt a facilitative pedagogy with more responsibility for learning transferring to students who were required to become actively engaged in the learning process. Issues of organisation and resourcing also had to be addressed by academic and administrative staff.

In sharing some of our experiences we hope to help you avoid some of the difficulties which can creep up unawares as you develop and implement a problem-based curriculum. The book aims to provide practical help with the organisational issues that require to be addressed in PBL. With this in mind we have adopted an interactive approach to the design of the text, which allows you to stop, consider and reflect on the essential issues while reading this text. While we do provide suggestions on how to solve some of the key issues, we would encourage you to engage in the activities to help you conceptualise your own thinking and stage of development in relation to PBL within your own organisation. This 'distance learning' approach, although not a direct mirror of the PBL approach to learning, does challenge you to stop and think, and come up with your own ideas and solutions to the issues which we feel are the key to ensuring the successful development and ultimate introduction of PBL into the curriculum.

Chapter 1 sets out the agenda for this publication, introducing the relevance of PBL in modern professional education in general and in particular to the recent developments in nursing and midwifery education. The common terminology associated with PBL is defined. This chapter provides a guide on getting the most from this text to enhance your understanding of the current issues relevant to introducing PBL into a nursing curriculum. Chapter 2 reviews the development of PBL and outlines the PBL approach to learning and teaching. It explores the current position of nurse education and provides support for PBL as a strategy which meets the needs of a profession that requires its graduates to be 'fit for practice' and have developed 'lifelong learning skills'. In this context we examine key aspects of preparing for the introduction of PBL, developing the student's learning styles to ensure a match with the requirement of a student undertaking PBL and the key role played by the facilitator in ensuring the success of PBL once introduced into the curriculum.

Chapter 3 explores the nature of the 'problem' within PBL and provides insight on building up problem-based scenarios within nurse education. Suggestions on the types of material that can be used to 'trigger' students learning are included. The following Chapter 4 discusses and debates the practical issues that need to be addressed when considering introducing PBL into the curriculum. These include the size of PBL teams, selecting of PBL team membership, the process of team building, student roles in PBL and the match between PBL and the objectives of the programme. If these key issues are ignored or not taken sufficiently into account in the planning stages, then implementation and ongoing curricular problems may surface as the programme evolves, '*forewarned is forearmed*'. If little thought is given to these issues then PBL will fail to fulfil its potential to prepare students for the realities of nursing practice, with students being disadvantaged during their educational journey. It is essential that curriculum planners take cognisance of these issues, as a considered approach to PBL implementation will ensure your curriculum is fit for purpose and fully prepares nurses for the demands of clinical practice.

In Chapter 5 we invite all readers to assume the role of a nursing student and to work through the PBL process for themselves. Working through a scenario in this way, although without the input from a team, will help you gain increased awareness of how the PBL process works in action. It can be difficult to perceive how a short paragraph promotes learning. Chapter 5 will assist you to experience the activity for yourself. Chapter 6 examines the issue of 'critical thinking' as an essential requirement for nurses in the 21st century, and explores how a PBL approach to curriculum development will help ensure your students have the opportunity to develop this essential skill. The material presents issues related to facilitation, questioning and reflection, integrating fixed resource sessions into the curriculum and student organisation and presentation of material during a PBL session. It offers you the opportunity to consider how these key areas, if handled with skill, will enhance your students' educational journey and challenge them to become 'critical thinkers' ready to take nursing forward in the new millennium.

An opportunity to consider the elements that lead to student dissatisfaction with the PBL process is offered in Chapter 7. In particular the concepts of *disjunction* (feeling lost within the PBL process) and *frame factors* (issues not directly related to the purpose of the PBL team meeting but which detract the student from engaging fully within the PBL process) are considered. Poor management of these concepts by the facilitator can lead to a traumatic educational experience for both the student and the facilitator. Within this context we examine these concepts, along with institutional assessment strategies and the problem of non-participation of team members and/or poor attendance at PBL team meetings. It is essential that academic staff are adequately prepared to not only develop the PBL curriculum but also to deal with these 'real' issues related to on-the-ground implementation of PBL within the PBL team meeting. It is with this in mind that we deal with these practical issues which can make or break the PBL programme, offering some advice and guidance to allow these issues to be resolved in a positive pro-active way to enhance rather that detract form student learning.

The final chapter considers evaluation of the whole gamut of PBL, from the management of the PBL process, the performance of facilitators and students to the congruence of PBL within the curriculum. Evaluation of any new development is essential to justify its continued use and to identify both good practice and the need for improvement. We believe that PBL has much to offer nurse education. However as it is a resource-intensive strategy, ongoing evaluation is necessary to ensure that it does not become routine and thus poorly implemented.

KAY WILKIE AND IAIN BURNS
University of Dundee

Acknowledgements

Robert Rankin for drawing the cartoon.

1

Introduction

Introduction

This book is designed to assist teachers of nursing and their students to gain increased understanding and skill in the application of problem-based learning (PBL) in nurse education. The first chapter presents the PBL strategy and its value in the education of nurses. Using examples, the PBL process is introduced in subsequent chapters with assessment related to PBL and suggestions for evaluating PBL comprising the final chapters.

Background

Problem-based learning is a learning/teaching strategy that encourages students to develop self-directed learning and critical thinking skills. In contrast to traditional curricula where the material to be taught is organised according to subject, problem-based curricula are designed around a series of 'problems' that students have to resolve. In the problems students are asked to consider patient/client focused situations where there is a need for a nursing intervention or interventions that will improve the situation for the patient or client. PBL differs from problem-solving or case-based learning in that students are presented with the situation prior to the learning taking place, rather than the more usual format where students are taught about a subject and then asked to apply what they have learned to the given situation. In PBL students are expected to engage with the material. Students work together in small groups to identify the issues in the situation which need to be addressed, decide what they already know and what they need to learn in order to suggest and justify how the situation can be improved. Learning is very much in the control of the students. Teaching staff act as facilitators to promote discussion and provide assistance, but they do not run the group as formal tutorials. Most nursing and midwifery programmes also include taught sessions such as lectures and other learning opportunities, for example clinical skills or laboratory workshops which complement the learning undertaken for the PBL situation. In addition a range of resources including libraries, computer assisted learning programmes, the Internet and clinical experts can be used to assist learning.

Group working requires the development of team-working/managing skills. This book aims to help with the development of these skills. PBL differs from other types of small group work in that the material to be learned and the running of the session are largely under that control of the students. This book considers issues in PBL from the point of view of both the student and the facilitator. Students participating in PBL will be expected to chair or act as scribe for the group at some point and thus take on part of the facilitator role. Facilitators will find that insight into the student perspective will assist in understanding the dynamics of the PBL group.

The value of PBL in nurse education

PBL has been widely used in medical education since the 1960s and is currently a major learning strategy for a variety of vocational programmes ranging from architecture and law to occupational therapy. PBL is an attractive strategy for teachers of programmes that have a practice element as learning is contextualised and integrated. Students are presented with situations drawn from practice that reflect reality and likely to be encountered by students during clinical placements. Organisations such as the World Health Organisation (WHO) and the World Bank recommend the use of PBL in programmes that prepare health care professionals as the use of PBL allows the programme to reflect the health care problems prevalent in the areas in which students will work.

The introduction of PBL into UK nurse education began with undergraduate and post-registration programmes where the number of students was small. Interest in PBL as a suitable strategy for nurse education increased throughout the 1990s with September 1997 seeing the introduction of problem-based pre-registration diploma programmes by three UK institutions. The desire for a different strategy in the education of British nurses, like the original McMaster Experiment, lay in dissatisfaction with the existing programmes. Dissatisfaction not only among nurse teachers, but also among practitioners who felt that the diploma programmes introduced in 1992, the so-called Project 2000 initiative, had failed to produce the expected 'knowledgeable doers' promised by the United Kingdom Central Council for Nursing, Midwifery and Health Visiting (UKCC, 1986). Increased teaching of subjects such as psychology, sociology and health policies in the Project 2000 programmes led to overcrowding in the curriculum with a subsequent shift to surface learning by students (Glen, 1995). This, coupled with the decline in opportunities for clinical practice resulting from changes in the NHS, brought allegations that curricula lacked sufficient integration of theory with practice in the clinical setting (Hislop *et al.*, 1996). These claims were followed by a series of reports that raised concerns over the ability of Project 2000 to equip nurses for practice (Walsh, 1997; Scott, 1997; Runciman *et al.*, 1998). The problems of theory overload, dwindling practice opportunities and lack of theory and practice linkage were compounded by Government initiatives, such as those outlined in The Learning Age (1998), to promote lifelong learning and transferable skills. As views on how best to prepare nurses tend to reflect the prevailing socio-political climate as well as professional interests, these elements were added to the mix. The Dearing and Garrick reports (1997) emphasised the use of flexible, self-directed approaches to learning in preference to the traditional teacher-centred, subject-based methods. This emphasis was echoed by the Report of the UKCC Commission for Nursing and Midwifery Education (1999) which responded to the issues outlined above and to many others, including attrition rates, entry requirements and relationships with Higher Education Institutions (HEIs) and services providers, with a series of recommendations whose main focus was Fitness for Practice. The use of PBL was recommended as a strategy that would foster interpersonal and practice skills and thus make the best use of practice placements. Learning was again highlighted as a lifelong activity.

rather than the teachers' teaching. Teachers should curb their enthusiasm and allow students to make their own discoveries, if students, in turn, were to become enthused.

In the UK the Diploma in Nursing programmes introduced under the Project 2000 initiative in the late 1980s/early 1990s have been criticised by the profession for failing to produce nurses who are 'Fit for Practice' (Runciman *et al.*, 1998; Scott, 1997). Changes to the organisation of the National Health Service throughout the 1990s have resulted in a loss of placements for nursing students coupled with a decrease in the number of qualified staff available to act as preceptors or mentors (Glen and Nicol, 1999). These problems have been compounded by the 'New Labour' government schemes to increase the numbers of nurses and midwives by recruiting more entrants into nursing and midwifery programmes without a corresponding increase in placements, especially in community settings. A new approach to nursing and midwifery programmes is needed to provide students with an educational experience that is relevant to future practice and that prepares them to deal with the constantly changing climate of health care in the 21st century.

Fitness for Practice (1999), the UKCC Report on Nursing and Midwifery Education, recommends PBL as a means of integrating theory with practice. Through the use of carefully created scenarios or 'problems', PBL sets learning in the context in which it will be needed in the clinical environment. The strategy allows a high degree of flexibility. Issues that are topical or changes in treatment can quickly be placed in the curriculum with minimal disruption and without waiting for a programme re-write. Students often contribute new knowledge on topics. PBL integrates material from different subject areas and applies them to the nursing situation, for example, a problem which centres on the nursing interventions required by an injured child arriving at an accident and emergency department will require not only learning about wound assessment, dressings and aseptic technique but also the physiology of healing, communicating with children, accidental and non-accidental injury and giving advice to parents. Students are expected to provide the research-based evidence to justify their choice of intervention, to question and challenge their decisions and to develop critical thinking skills. The identification of what knowledge is needed and the ability to resource, learn and defend nurse education increased throughout the 1990s with September 1997 seeing the introduction of problem-based pre-registration diploma programmes by three UK institutions. The desire for a different strategy in the education of British nurses, like the original McMaster Experiment, lay in dissatisfaction with the existing programmes. Dissatisfaction not only among nurse teachers, but also among practitioners who felt that the diploma programmes introduced in 1992, the so-called Project 2000 initiative, had failed to produce the expected 'knowledgeable doers' promised by the United Kingdom Central Council for Nursing, Midwifery and Health Visiting (UKCC, 1986). Increased teaching of subjects such as psychology, sociology and health policies in the Project 2000 programmes led to overcrowding in the curriculum with a subsequent shift to surface learning by students (Glen, 1995). This, coupled with the decline in opportunities for clinical practice resulting from changes in the NHS, brought allegations that curricula lacked sufficient integration of theory with practice in the clinical setting (Hislop *et al.*, 1996). These claims were followed by a series of reports that raised concerns over the ability of Project 2000 to equip nurses for practice (Walsh, 1997; Scott, 1997; Runciman *et al.*, 1998). The problems of theory overload, dwindling practice opportunities and lack of theory and practice linkage were compounded by Government initiatives, such as those outlined in The Learning Age (1998), to promote lifelong learning and transferable skills. As views on how best to prepare nurses tend to reflect the prevailing socio-political climate as well as professional interests, these elements were added to the mix. The Dearing and Garrick reports (1997) emphasised the use of flexible, self-directed approaches to learning in preference to the traditional teacher-centred, subject-based methods. This emphasis was echoed by the Report of the UKCC Commission for Nursing and Midwifery Education (1999) which responded to the issues outlined above and to many others, including attrition rates, entry requirements and relationships with Higher Education Institutions (HEIs) and services providers, with a series of recommendations whose main focus was Fitness for Practice. The use of PBL was recommended as a strategy that would foster interpersonal and practice skills and thus make the best use of practice placements. Learning was again highlighted as a lifelong activity.

Although the employment situation for nurses began to improve in the late 1990s, the nursing workplace continued to be subject to constant change, thus continuing to require flexibility in its employees. The National Board for Nursing, Midwifery and Health Visiting for Scotland (NBS) expected nursing students to develop transferable skills through collaborative and peer activities, participatory, interactive learning and inter-disciplinary learning situations in which they were not only expected to learn, but also to enjoy the learning experience enough to continue learning through life (Hickie, 1998). The move into higher education brought pressures to increase the academic level of the initial preparation programme to that of degree, while practitioners insisted that courses must not become increasingly academic and create practitioners who are not able cope with, in the words of Schön, 'the complexity, uncertainty, instability, uniqueness and value conflicts perceived as central to the world of professional practice' (Schön, 1987, p. 16). Given the demands on nurse education at a time when educationalists felt scapegoated for nursing's wider problems and burdened by the demands of academe, it was unsurprising that PBL, with its claims of active, contextualised learning which promotes critical thinking and problem-solving while enhancing communication skills and team-working, appeared an attractive strategy for nurse education.

Considerations in implementing PBL

While PBL offers several apparent benefits, which seem to meet the demands on nurse education to produce a practitioner fit for 21st century healthcare, it also carries several drawbacks. Feletti (1993) argued that the hypothetical-deductive nature of problem-based learning was not particularly suited to nurses or their education. He claimed that nursing students overall, tend to be less academically able than medical students are, and thus may be less confident in discussion and less competent in self-directed learning. He suggested that this may be linked to the number of women in nursing, indicating that women's knowledge and preferred learning styles were less suited to PBL. As very few research studies address the influence of gender in PBL and the research into women's ways of learning is itself inconclusive (Hofer and

Pintrich, 1997), there appears to be little basis for this statement. Feletti (1993) also claimed that the 'messy problems' encountered in nursing do not lend themselves to solution through PBL. This statement is countered by work by Sadlo (1995) which suggested that PBL is useful in learning about these 'messy problems' as it allows for integration of material and discussion around real situations which are seldom clear cut. Feletti's third argument against PBL in nurse education stated that as there are considerably more nursing students than medical students, PBL may not be feasible because of staff resource implications. This point is arguable as Schools of Nursing currently tend to have more full-time members of staff than Medical Schools who traditionally work with large numbers of honorary lecturers. Schools of Nursing may, in fact, be better placed to operate problem-based curricula.

Despite the reservations of Feletti about the unsuitability of PBL as a strategy for nurse education, the biggest potential hindrance to adopting PBL, not only in nurse education, but in other disciplines, is the fear that introducing PBL will result in teachers losing both their teaching and subject expertise and thus their status as teachers. The basis for this fear lies in teachers' pedagogical beliefs. Successful facilitation of PBL depends on teachers possessing a concept of learning, and hence teaching, that is student empowering, that believes in the students' ability to learn and that perceives knowledge as a changing and shared product. The concept does not hold that teachers own the knowledge that they transmit to students or that there is a collection of 'right' answers to be learned and reproduced. Unless teachers espouse and apply such concepts, facilitation will not be effective in producing the benefits claimed for PBL.

Rogers and Freiberg (1994) pointed out that being a facilitator requires a special perspective on life. Facilitators are people who place learners' needs and interests first, an attribute recognised and appreciated by most students. PBL is claimed as being enjoyable for both students and teachers – a view supported by Albanese and Mitchell (1993) who commented that PBL appeared to be more successful when delivered by a small group of enthusiastic lecturers rather than by everyone in the Faculty. The enthusiasm in the Albanese and Mitchell study was for PBL. Elton (2000) suggested that in a problem-based learning curriculum the enthusiasm for the subject should come from the students' learning rather than the teachers' teaching. Teachers should curb their enthusiasm and allow students to make their own discoveries, if students, in turn, were to become enthused.

In the UK the Diploma in Nursing programmes introduced under the Project 2000 initiative in the late 1980s/early 1990s have been criticised by the profession for failing to produce nurses who are 'Fit for Practice' (Runciman *et al.*, 1998; Scott, 1997). Changes to the organisation of the National Health Service throughout the 1990s have resulted in a loss of placements for nursing students coupled with a decrease in the number of qualified staff available to act as preceptors or mentors (Glen and Nicol, 1999). These problems have been compounded by the 'New Labour' government schemes to increase the numbers of nurses and midwives by recruiting more entrants into nursing and midwifery programmes without a corresponding increase in placements, especially in community settings. A new approach to nursing and midwifery programmes is needed to provide students with an educational experience that is relevant to future practice and that prepares them to deal with the constantly changing climate of health care in the 21st century.

Fitness for Practice (1999), the UKCC Report on Nursing and Midwifery Education, recommends PBL as a means of integrating theory with practice. Through the use of carefully created scenarios or 'problems', PBL sets learning in the context in which it will be needed in the clinical environment. The strategy allows a high degree of flexibility. Issues that are topical or changes in treatment can quickly be placed in the curriculum with minimal disruption and without waiting for a programme re-write. Students often contribute new knowledge on topics. PBL integrates material from different subject areas and applies them to the nursing situation, for example, a problem which centres on the nursing interventions required by an injured child arriving at an accident and emergency department will require not only learning about wound assessment, dressings and aseptic technique but also the physiology of healing, communicating with children, accidental and non-accidental injury and giving advice to parents. Students are expected to provide the research-based evidence to justify their choice of intervention, to question and challenge their decisions and to develop critical thinking skills. The identification of what knowledge is needed and the ability to resource, learn and defend their actions, assists students to develop the skills needed for life-long learning – a transferable skill essential to keeping abreast of the constant developments in health care. In addition to skills related to learning, PBL fosters communication skills. Students are required to explain rationales for action clearly to their peers; they need to develop team working and negotiating skills to ensure that work is distributed equitably. The PBL seminars provide a safe environment to test interview skills and hone questioning techniques. Nursing tasks such as assessment and care planning can also be developed through the use of PBL.

PBL terminology

Like many other areas, PBL has a language of its own where everyday words have a meaning specific to PBL. To add to the confusion not all institutions that have adopted a PBL approach in their programmes, use the same terms in the same way. Even the term 'Problem-based Learning' is contentious. Many people, particularly those who work in the health care professions, dislike the word 'problem' which is perceived as having negative connotations. There is a reluctance to label patients/clients as being problematic. Additionally it is sometimes stated that the so-called problem is not, in fact, a problem. The situation is acceptable; it is simply in need of some improvement. Some institutions, therefore, have chosen to label the strategy 'enquiry-based learning (EBL)', 'context-based learning (CBL)', 'task-based learning (TBL)' or 'case-based learning (CBL)'. Sometimes these strategies can be identified as being 'problem-based', however sometimes the strategy is more akin to discovery learning or problem-solving rather than PBL.

It is important to remember that the 'problem' is a situation that creates learning needs for the student. The problem lies in the students' lack of knowledge about the situation, a difficulty that is often perceived as being easily remedied by someone who knows the answer, namely the teacher. Margetson (1994) points out that there is not only a problem with 'problem' but also an issue with the term 'based' as the base for learning is the issues generated by the students and the material used to reach a solution rather than the problem. PBL was the term originally used and although there is much discussion about its accuracy, it generally continues to be used for strategies in which small groups of students generate their own learning needs from an unfamiliar situation.

Problem-based learning may be viewed only as a strategy which adheres fairly rigidly to the outline propounded by Barrows (1986) where students in groups of four or five work through the set problem in a hypothetical-deductive manner. In nurse education in general, there are simply too many students for PBL group size to be restricted to 4 or 5. Ten–twelve is a more likely size for the PBL group, although some Schools of Nursing and Midwifery report PBL style strategies with groups of 20–25 students. Gatterman (1997) reported on PBL-style techniques used successfully with a large student group (approx. 150). Gatterman pointed out however, that with large groups the interaction and discussion is limited. When the students are sub-divided into small teams to undertake the work, some of the PBL characteristics are lost.

Barrows (1986) pointed out that there are innumerable permutations and combinations of PBL. PBL has the attributes of using small groups of students, presents the problem before related issues are taught, is student-centred, uses adult learning principles, and promotes critical thinking. Learning strategies that have most of these attributes may be classed as 'problem-based'. The process of nursing assessment and diagnoses differ from that of medical diagnosis, thus there may be less need for a hypothetical deductive mode. The creation of a nursing action plan based on evidence-based practice may be more applicable. Vernon and Blake (1993, p. 560) undertook a study of problem-based undergraduate medical programmes and came to the conclusion that PBL is:

> A complex mixture of a general teaching philosophy, learning objectives and goals and faculty attitudes and values all of which are difficult to regulate and often are not well defined in research reports.

The terminology used for the actual pragmatics of PBL varies from institution to institution and even from programme to programme.

PBL glossary

PBL group or team: the students who work together on the problems. Usually the School or Department of Nursing and Midwifery allocates students randomly to PBL groups. An attempt may be made to mix students according to gender, entrance route, age or educational experience. Some Schools mix students from different branches of nursing for PBL in the Foundation Programme, while others prefer PBL groups to be single branch from day one. Students may be allowed to choose PBL teams later in the programme (see Chapter 4).

Entwistle (1987) and Savin-Baden (2000) discuss the merits of the term 'team' versus 'group'. Groups are viewed as being less formal, members share a common interest and there is an option about becoming or remaining in the group. Teams, on the other hand, are seen as being created for a specific purpose; members may have no common interest other than the team's purpose and membership is not optional. Some Schools refer to student groupings for PBL as teams rather than groups for these reasons. It is argued that this mirrors the situation in practice. Nursing and/or multidisciplinary team members seldom choose to work together and often have nothing in common apart from work. The argument continues to suggest that PBL offers the opportunity for students to develop team-working skills in a controlled, safe environment. This argument can be countered by the fact that all students in the PBL team are of equal status with each one's view carrying the same weight, a situation that rarely occurs in practice. The term 'PBL team' will be used throughout this book.

PBL teams may be the same throughout the programme. Once students are allocated to teams, they stay in them. Other institutions may change the teams between the Foundation and Branch parts of the programme. Sometimes teams are changed with each new problem or in every term.

Facilitator: as the name suggests this is someone who promotes, enhances, encourages and eases the way for the team during PBL. Other terms used may include tutor or leader. Although this person is usually a member of teaching staff, facilitators may be clinical staff with a specialist expertise, lecturer/practitioners or senior students. There is much debate as to whether facilitators need an in-depth knowledge of the subject under discussion or whether good facilitation skills are preferable. Ideally facilitators would possess both. Given the current situation in nurse education with rising numbers of students and a shortage of qualified teaching staff, this is not always possible. What is essential is that

PBL packages are compiled by subject experts (cf. Chapter 3). Margetson (1997) suggests that good PBL facilitators are simply good teachers. Vernon (1995) found that teachers who were enthusiastic about the technique were rated highly by students but that not all faculty staff enjoyed PBL or wanted to be involved in it. The work of Dolmans and Schidt *et al.* (1994) and de Grave *et al.* (1999) into student evaluation of facilitators suggested that not every faculty member would automatically be a satisfactory PBL facilitator. As students progress through a problem-based programme, there is a perception that their need for a facilitator should decrease as they become increasingly self-motivated and self-directed.

Trigger: 'triggers' are the material which is used to stimulate discussion. Triggers come in a wide variety from patient notes to cartoons or photographs. They may give in-depth patient detail or only the outline of the issue (see Chapter 3).

Situation: the situation may form part or the entire trigger or it may be additional to the trigger and provide information about the nurse and what is expected of her in relation to the trigger.

Scenario: sometimes used interchangeably with 'trigger', sometimes used to include the trigger and the situation.

Package: may also be referred to as a facilitator pack(age), a situation improvement pack(age) (SIP), patient/client case, PBL pack/material, scenario or simply the 'PBL'. This includes all of the material needed for any particular session. It includes the trigger material, the situation and facilitator's guidelines. It may also include some additional material related to the trigger such as blood results, doctors' letters and some resource material for example reference lists, web sites, experts willing to be contacted and key articles. The facilitator's guidelines contain learning outcomes related to both content and the PBL process; hints on pacing; expected student responses in relation to knowledge, skills and attitudes; possible questions and resources (see Chapter 3).

Fixed resource: in PBL this term applies to resources such as lectures, workshops, clinical skills sessions, which have been organised to support the topic, being discussed in the PBL seminar. Obviously it is beyond the remit of this book to organise resources, which are 'fixed', however you will be given references and 'unfixed' resource material.

Scribe: person (student) appointed by the team in rotation to record discussion and issues raised.

Chairperson: appointed by the team in rotation to steer group discussion and clarify issues. May also simultaneously act as scribe.

Getting the most from this book

The book aims to help you get the best from PBL through understanding the PBL process and making it work for you. The book may be read from cover to cover, but you will probably find it more useful to dip in and out of the various chapters as their topics occur within PBL in your own programmes. Each chapter deals with a different aspect of PBL. Some aspects you will encounter immediately. Others, such as disjunction, you may not encounter until part way through the programme. Each chapter contains examples and activities for you to work through. As PBL is a team strategy, you may find it useful to work on the activities with two or three other colleagues.

The book does not contain the content required in a pre-registration nursing/midwifery, or indeed, any other, programme. Rather it provides hints on how to manage PBL and thus to develop the lifelong learning skills required by nurses/midwives in today's health care environment.

References

Albanese, M A and Mitchell, S (1993) Problem-based Learning: A review of Literature on its Outcomes and Implementation Issues, *Academic Medicine*, **68**(1): 52–81.

Barrows, H S (1986) A Taxonomy of problem-based learning methods, *Medical Education*, **20**: 481–6.

De Grave, W, Dolmans, D H J M and van der Vleuten, C P M (1999) Profiles of effective tutors in problem-based learning: scaffolding student learning, *Medical Education*, **33**: 901–6.

Department for Education and Employment (1998) *The Learning Age: A Renaissance for a New Britain*: London, HMSO.

Dolmans, D H J M, Wolfhagen, I A P, Schmidt, H G and van der Vleuten, C P M (1994) A rating scale for tutor evaluation in a problem-based curriculum: validity and reliability, *Medical Education*, **28**: 550–8.

Elton, L (2000) Turning Academics into Teachers: a discourse on love, *Teaching in Higher Education*, **5**(2): 257–60.

Entwistle, N (1983) Understanding Classroom Learning, London: Hodder and Stoughton.

Feletti, G (1993) Inquiry-based and Problem-based Learning: How similar are these approaches to nursing and medical education? *Higher Education Research and Development*, **12**(2): 143–56.

Gatterman, M I (1997) Teaching chiropractic principles through patient-centred problems, *Journal of the Canadian Chiropractic Association*, **41**(1): 27–35.

Glen, S (1995) Developing Critical Thinking in Higher Education, *Nurse Education Today*, **15**: 170–6.

Glen, S and Nicol, M (1999) *Clinical Skills in Nursing: Return of the Practical Room?* Macmillan – now Palgrave Macmillan: Basingstoke.

Hickie, S (1998) *Information Base on Arrangements which support the Development of Clinical Practice in Pre-Registration Nursing Programmes in Scotland*, National Board for Nursing, Midwifery and Health Visiting for Scotland: Edinburgh.

Hislop, S, Inglis, B, Cope, P, Stoddart, B and McIntosh, C (1996) Situating Theory in Practice: Student Views of Theory and Practice in Project 2000 Nursing Programmes, *Journal of Advanced Nursing*, **23**: 171–7.

Hofer, B K and Pintrich, P (1997) The Development of Epistemological Theories: Beliefs About Knowledge and Knowing and Their Relation to Learning, *Review of Educational Research*, **67**(1): 88–140.

Margetson, D (1994) Beginning with the essentials: why problem-based learning begins with problems, *Education for Health*, **9**(1): 61–70.

Margetson, D (1997) *Wholeness and educative learning: the question of problems in changing to problem-based learning.* Paper Changing to PBL Conference, Brunel University, September 1997.

National Committee of Enquiry into Higher Education, Dearing, R (Chairman) (1997) *Higher Education in the Learning Society*, NCHIE.

National Committee of Enquiry into Higher Education, Garrick, R (Chairman, Scottish Committee) (1997) *Higher Education in the Learning Society: Report of the Scottish Committee*, NCHIE.

Rogers, C and Freiberg, H J (1994) *Freedom to Learn*, 3rd edition, New York: Merill.

Runciman, P, Dewar, B and Gouldbourne, A (1998) *Employers' Needs and the Skills of Newly Qualified Staff Project 2000 Nurses*, Queen Margaret College: Edinburgh.

Sadlo, G (1995) Problem-based Learning, *Tertiary Education News*, **5**(6): 8–10.

Savin-Baden, M (2000) *Problem-based Learning in Higher Education: Untold Stories*, The Society for Research into Higher Education and Open University Press: Buckingham.

Schön, D (1987) *Educating the Reflective Practitioner*, London: Jossey-Bass.

Scott, G (1997) Diploma Nurses Need Extra Year to Gain Clinical Skills, *Nursing Standard*, **12**(1): 5.

UKCC (1999) *Fitness for Practice*, Report of the UKCC Commission for Nursing and Midwifery Education, Chairman Sir Leonard Peach, UKCC: London.

Vernon, D T A and Blake, R L (1993) Does Problem-based Learning Work?: A Meta-Analysis of Educative Research, *Academic Medicine*, **68**(7): 550–63.

Vernon, D T A (1995) Attitudes and Opinions of Faculty Tutors about Problem-based Learning, *Academic Medicine*, **70**(3): 216–23.

Walsh, M (1997) Accountability and Intuition: Justifying Nursing Practice, *Nursing Standard*, **11**(23): 39–41.

WHO (1993) *Increasing the Relevance of Education for Health Professionals*, Report of a WHO study group on problem-solving education for the health professionals. WHO Technical Report Series 838: Geneva.

World Bank (1993) World Development Report 1993: *Investing in Health*, Oxford University Press for the World Bank: Oxford.

2

An Introduction to Problem-based Learning

Introduction

This chapter will explore not only the development of PBL but also address some of the key issues that need to be examined when considering a PBL approach to curriculum development.

Nursing has a duty to provide society with skilled and educated practitioners. It is therefore essential that nursing curricula reflect this and, although not wholly skills-led, take cognisance of the real world of practice. This will ensure that the knowledge and skills developed by students leads to compassionate and skilled care in clinical practice. The nurse of the 21st century according to Bevis and Watson (1989, p. 1), must 'be more responsive to societal needs, more successful in humanising the highly techno-logical milieus of health care, more caring and compassionate, more insightful about ethical and moral issues, more creative, more capable of critical thinking, and better able to bring schol-arly approaches to client problems and issues'. Nurses therefore need to be prepared to become 'life long learners' who have been exposed to 'innovative' learning strategies which prepare them, not only to function effectively in the current clinical setting but also to be able to take nursing practice forward to benefit both nursing and the society it serves.

Nurse education programmes at all academic levels must be cost effective, innovative and up to date, and also produce the desired outcome, in terms of nurses who are 'fit for practice' and ready to meet the challenges of an ever changing health service. It is there-fore not surprising that there has been a great deal of debate about how to prepare nurses for practice. Alavi (1995) stressed that in order to move forward in the development of the nursing curriculum, it is neccesary for nurse educators to have considered a key question and have arrived at an answer. The question Alavi (1995, p. 1) suggested must be answered was: 'What kind of curriculum will help students to become competent professionals?'.

In answering this question and developing nursing curricula educationalists and practitioners of nursing must identify, 'what knowledge and skills do nurses need to practice?', 'how do we help students gain the appropriate knowledge and skills for effective practice?' and 'how do we facilitate the development of life-long learning skills in our students?' It is essential in considering the answer to these issues that nurse education takes cognisance of 'the messy, real world of nursing practice' (Miller, 1985, p. 420). Problem-based Learning (PBL) is offered by many educationalists as a solution to some of these problems within professional education. Alavi (1995) suggested that PBL allows the integration of theory and practice through the use of real problem situations within the curriculum.

Problem-based learning

PBL was developed within the medical curriculum at the Case Western Reserve University in the United States during the late 1950s and McMaster University in Canada during the 1960s. From these institutions it spread within medicine and related areas world-wide during the 1970s and 1980s (Boud and Feletti, 1997). According to Boud and Feletti (1997) it is a model of adult education that is more than simply exposing students to a series of lectures and tutorials within a traditional curriculum. PBL is a method that allows the students to explore what Boud and Feletti (1997, p. 2) term 'real life' situations, with emphasis on problem solving and team-work in developing educational skills which will enable them to cope with an ever changing world where lifelong learning is essential.

It has been recognised that in many cases educationalists in all fields have been 'hanging on to curricula which have lost their point' (Margetson, 1994, p. 5). Similarly the World Health Organisation has pointed out that the education of health professionals does not always meet societal needs (WHO, 1993). They went on to advocate the widespread introduction of PBL into health professional education. This was in part due to the growing body of research and literature which provided and continues to provide evidence of the value of PBL curricula in the education of health care professionals. The literature indicates that there are advantages in utilising a PBL approach. Alavi (1995) found that students exposed to PBL had a more rewarding and useful clinical experience, while Doring *et al.* (1995) saw PBL as a way of fully involving students in the process of education. This process ensures that the students benefit from developing deeper knowledge rather than a surface approach to learning which depends on rote learning and skimming the surface of certain concepts within the educational process (Margetson, 1994). These concepts were explored in-depth by Marton and Saljo (1984). In their work they clearly identified that deeper learning requires the student to uncover meaning in learning while surface learning allows the student to adopt a rote learning strategy. It is essential that in preparing students for the demands of clinical practice that they are engaged in 'deep processing' and not surface learning as they are required to understand the meaning behind learning to ensure they can apply knowledge in clinical practice (Coles, 1997, p. 314).

However, one of the biggest challenges facing educationalists is 'what is important enough to be curriculum?' (MacDonald, 1991, p. 101). On the face of it this seems to be an easy question to answer. Boud and Feletti (1991) however, would argue that this question has not been answered in many traditional lecture based programmes, with an over reliance on subjects against the development of inquiry skills, a failure to deal with the issues faced by students in professional practice and poor development of team-working. Allied to this is the continual development of new knowledge, and the growing belief that it is not possible to include everything in the curriculum, even though as Ryan (1993) recognises there is often a demand for lecturers to cover all possible aspects of content. Traditional programmes according to Sadlo *et al.* (1994) therefore concentrate on knowledge gathering and not on the knowledge needed for practice, leading to an overloading of the curriculum and the development of surface learning as opposed to deep learning (Ramsden, 1991; Margetson, 1994). This may be one of the reasons why, even with a major educational change in the 1990s as a result of Project 2000, there was still a reliance on traditional teaching methods within nursing curricula which did not always prepare students for practice (McIntosh *et al.*, 1997; Runciman *et al.*, 1998). Nursing has been presented with a unique opportunity to remedy this situation with the development of new curricula, under the guidance of the UKCC's 1999 document 'Fitness for Practice'. In adopting a PBL model for curriculum design, the students are presented with a 'problem situation'. The emphasis is on encouraging the students to use their existing knowledge, a deficiency of traditional passive teaching methods (Amos and White, 1998), and explore 'what needs to be known to address and improve a particular situation' (Boud and Feletti, 1997, p. 16).

Nursing is a practice based profession, therefore the knowledge gained must help nurses engage in and develop their practice. Nurse education must, as Townsend (1990, p. 61) suggested, be based on a curriculum that is 'grounded in and derived from that practice'. PBL is advocated as a model of adult education which allows this to happen. It is a method that enables students to explore what Boud and Feletti (1997, p. 2) term 'real life' situations, with the emphasis on problem solving and team-work. Students therefore are able to develop educational and practical skills which will enable them to cope with an ever-changing world where lifelong learning is essential.

PBL is seen as a way to encouraging deeper learning which is relevant to practice. Doring *et al.* (1995) see PBL as a way of ensuring that students become fully involved in the learning process. Townsend (1990) amongst others, pointed out that as the problem situations or triggers utilised within the PBL component of the curriculum are drawn from practice, the solutions or knowledge required to deal with the issues must therefore be directly related to the practice situation. This means that the PBL offers a more integrated approach to learning and the learning which takes place will enable the student to approach care delivery in a holistic manner (Williams, 1998). This is supported by Bawden (1997, p. 326), in discussing PBL within a curricula for professional agriculturists. He noted that in a traditional curricula there is a 'fragmentation of effort' which works against the development of the skills needed for today's professional practice. PBL, on the other hand, ensures that the students 'learn how to improve situations across an enormous range of complexity, through their involvement in real world projects' (Bawden, 1997, p. 331).

The problem-based learning process

A basic premise of PBL is that through the context of 'problem solving' learning takes place. This according to Barrows and Tamblyn (1980) is a process which reflects everyday life both in the workplace and in our everyday experience.

Activity 2.1
Consider how you resolve or meet challenges presented to you on a day to day basis.

Commentary 2.1
You will have examined and asked yourself questions about real life issues from both your personal and professional life. This may have included issues related to planning an annual holiday or introducing a new innovation in practice. Whatever the 'scenario' you are faced with, learning takes place either concisely or unconsciously in order to move forward and meet the challenges triggered by life events which need resolved.

PBL is a process within education that attempts to mirror the real life situation in a simulated and safe educational environment. As a result of this process real life knowledge and skills are developed through the process of working towards an understanding of the problems/ challenges presented.

Educationalists who argue that this is only another form of group work, miss a key point in the structure of the PBL process. The 'problem' or 'challenge' presented in the scenario is positioned at the beginning of the learning process rather than after the student has had their mind filled with the lecturers' solutions through the traditional teaching and learning methods such as lectures and tutorials. This format of facilitating learning does not, however, seek to undermine traditional methods of teaching but ensures that strategies are selected and used for the purpose of meaningful learning which is relevant to clinical practice and develops the students as a self autonomous 'lifelong learner'.

Activity 2.2
Consider how you would feel if, before deciding on your annual holiday, the whole holiday plus the day to day itinerary was presented to you and was not open for negotiation.

Commentary 2.2
This may at first seem acceptable to many and would certainly make life easier. However, think again, how much autonomy does this give you in deciding on what you want from the holiday and how much control do you have on the outcome of this holiday?

For a student who is developing the skills and knowledge to work effectively in a complex and 'messy' world of practice it is no longer possible, if it ever was, to give a recipe that will see them through the challenges presented in practice. The 'knowledge' explosion aided by the internet makes it impossible for traditional teaching methods alone to prepare students for the real world of clinical practice.

Nursing requires its practitioners to develop knowledge and skills in order to not only deliver care but also to be innovative and develop key learning skills. It is therefore essential that the educational process engages the student as a active participant of knowledge/skills acquisition and not a passive recipient of knowledge.

The unique and 'messy' world of practice demands more of a nurse than simply following an instruction or a 'core care plan'. Not every situation encountered in practice will be linear in nature and students must have been exposed to an educational process which challenges them to explore care options. This will enable them to make decisions about nursing practice in a safe environment which allows them to learn how to resolve issues in the real world. Lecturers can no longer claim to have all the answers and must be prepared to be challenged, while students in the PBL process must be encouraged to 'contest the solution offered by the tutor; to value their own perspectives and their own voices enough in the learning process to argue their case' (Savin-Baden, 2000, p. 1). Since the introduction of Project 2000 students have been encouraged to be assertive and challenge 'the system', and act as the patients advocate. Biley and Smith (1998) support this and add that the new nurse must also be prepared to be an autonomous practitioner who is active in clinical decision making. This, according to Savin-Baden (2000, p. 1), may be difficult for students who have undertaken a traditional lecture based programme as, unlike PBL, the nature of teaching and learning in that environment may not have encouraged the student to engage in the deeper learning required to deal with and 'manage the ambiguities that prevail in professional life'.

Activity 2.3
Brainstorm all the key content areas which you consider important for a pre-registration curriculum in nursing.

Commentary 2.3
In considering this issue the easy part would be to outline the basic sub-ject areas, Nursing, Health, Biology, Psychology etc. The next part becomes more difficult. What do you include under each of these topic areas and what do you exclude? The demands on pre-registration edu-cation to serve all masters has in many instances led to an overloaded curriculum. This type of scenario leads to a broad brush approach to learning which according to Des Marchais (1993) encourages passive rote learning. This leaves the student little opportunity for in-depth study and the development in the study skills which will prepare them to engage in effective learning for current and future practice. The PBL approach to learning recognises that adult learners must be given responsibility for their learning and lectures become facilitators rather than the fountain of all knowledge.

In the PBL process the student is therefore central to the education process and is valued as a learning individual rather that a receptacle for the lecturer's knowledge. Students are encouraged to develop their own knowledge base, guided by the curriculum and the UKCC nursing competencies for registration rather than restricted by them (UKCC, 1999). PBL offers an alternative teach-ing method which has the potential to awaken the 'lifelong learner' in all our students.

Preparing for problem-based learning

The catalyst for introducing PBL into a nursing curriculum can vary from 'evangelism' common to much of the early introduction of, and research into PBL to a realisation that a practice based programme of education demands more active learning on the part of the student or the direct result of implementing the recommendations contained within 'Fitness for Practice' (UKCC, 1999). Whatever the initial stimulus, consideration must be given to preparing staff and students for a major shift in educational approach. This shift may challenge the educational philosophy of both staff and students, leading to potential casualties along the way. It is therefore essential that the challenges are met and overcome at the outset. This will ensure we embark on an educational journey that has the potential to enhance the education of the next generation of practitioners.

Activity 2.4
Brainstorm how PBL will challenge you as lecturer or student.

Commentary 2.4
Some of the issues you may have identified are:
Staff development, production of learning packs, how much PBL, how little PBL, PBL team size, PBL team selection, team facilitation, timetabling of PBL, timetabling of other teaching sessions, links to clinical practice, adapting students leaning styles to PBL, can I adapt either as a student or a lecturer to the demands of PBL.

Many of these issues and how to deal with them will be discussed in other chapters within this book, however at this point it is worth reflecting briefly on two key aspects which will affect the success or otherwise of PBL and your decision whether or not to explore further the unique learning opportunities offered by a PBL approach to nurse education. The issues which often cause most debate in the early stage of PBL development are related to the learning style of the students and the facilitation style of the lecturer. Successful PBL depends on students engaging in active learning facilitated by facilitators committed to the PBL approach to learning.

Learning styles

There has been a great deal of discussion in the literature with regards to learning style and the effect this has on students learning (Griggs and Griggs, 1998; Ramprogus, 1988; Cavanagh et al., 1994). The ability of students to learn and utilise what they have learned in practice can often be determined by a number of factors including their learning style (Ramprogus, 1988) and how they approach the learning process (Alexander, 1983; Vaughan, 1990). Students entering any programme of education can have varying learning styles (Cavanagh *et al.*, 1994).

This range of preferred learning styles of student nurses is not surprising when one considers the make-up of traditional entrants to 3 year pre-registration Higher Education Diploma/Degree Programmes in the United Kingdom. The age range of the students is from 17, the minimum age of entry into pre-registration nurse education, to students in their 40s and 50s, with their previous nursing backgrounds ranging from 'no nursing experience' to working as a 'registered nurses' on parts 2, 4, 6 and 7 of the UKCC Register. This is now a feature of today's pre-registration programmes both within the United Kingdom and throughout the Western World (Cavanagh and Coffin, 1994; Creedy and Alavi, 1997). This, in effect, means that nursing has to 'address a wider range of abilities, age, background and motivation for entry than any other discipline' (Creedy and Alavi, 1997, p. 219).

The choice of teaching methods utilised within a PBL curriculum must give the students the maximum opportunity to learn and, in particular, to begin to become competent 'lifelong learners'. This would be supported by most educationalists who recognise that we must use a variety of instructional methods to ensure all students' needs are catered for (Ramprogus, 1988). This allows students the opportunity to become familiar with various learning methods in order to improve their learning (Partridge, 1983) and develop into 'lifelong learners'. In recognising this, it is also important to take cognisance of the fact that PBL does challenge students in a unique way, due to the very nature of the fact that one starts with the 'problem' and not the knowledge to solve the 'problem'. As Ryan and Lyttle (1991) point out, they must become more active in their learning.

Those students whose learning styles are challenged by the very nature of PBL will therefore feel compromised. PBL does not offer any anonymity to students; they are expected to function and be active in the group, taking responsibility for their own learning (Ryan and Lyttle, 1991). Cavanagh and Coffin (1994, p. 109) point out that 'not all students will be comfortable with all learning approaches'. Within a programme that prepares students for clinical practice, how this is handled may well determine how the student perceives the learning process and how prepared they are for clinical practice. In light of this, it is often good practice for PBL facilitators to be aware of the individual student's learning style. This, according to Amos and White (1998), allows facilitators to take this into account in helping students to develop and progress within the PBL process, enabling them to develop 'life-long learning' skills. It is, however, encouraging for nursing to reflect on the small scale study carried out by Ramprogus (1988) who found that 52% of students entering pre-registration education were 'Allrounders' (Ramprogus, 1988, p. 62) and could adapt to different learning experiences and methods. This is essential if we are to encourage our students to meet the educational and clinical challenges presented in the new millenium.

It is also worth recognising that there is no place to hide in the real world of nursing and if we have students who want to hide during the educational process, are these the types of individuals who will make a difference in practice and provide society with expert professional nurses? We must expose students to the demands of active participative learning which challenges them to take reposibility for their own learning and ultimately their own clinical practice (see Chapters 5, 7 and 8).

Facilitation

The role of the facilitator in PBL is central to the success of a PBL curriculum (Happell, 1998; Schwartz *et al.*, 1997; Stern, 1997). According to Happell (1998, p. 364) the PBL facilitator's role is 'not to provide information in response to students questions but to assist them to discover what they need to know'. As Stern (1997) points out, this role is about giving the students guidance in order to allow them to take responsibility for their own learning.

In preparing to introduce PBL to any curriculum it is therefore essential that facilitation and the preparation of facilitators is high on the agenda of curriculum planners. Without preparation inappropriate facilitation can lead to ineffective PBL, inactive and passive learning which will not encourage independent 'deep learning'. Without clear guidance on facilitation and preparation of facilitators there is a danger that students will be exposed to tutor problems such as inexperience, tutor domination and negative attitudes (Rono, 1997).

Creedy and Alavi (1997) also emphasise the importance of skilful facilitation as being a key component of PBL, and recognise that eventually PBL teams should be self-directed, but not, in their opinion, until the third year of their pre-registration nursing programme rather than in the initial terms. It is also worth reflecting on the issue raised by Albanese and Mitchell (1993), when reviewing the literature on PBL. They recognised that PBL may be more successful when delivered by a small group of enthusiastic lecturers. It may be good practice to expose as many lecturers as possible to the PBL process, but it may be more beneficial to target committed enthusiasts to actually carry out the PBL facilitation, thus ensuring the students are truly facilitated through the PBL process (see Chapters 5, 6 and 7).

Conclusion

The UKCC recommendations contained within the report 'Fitness for Practice' (UKCC, 1999), offer nurse education the opportunity to review how it delivers pre-registration education. Within this context a PBL approach to curriculum design gives nursing an educational approach which has the potential to directly mirror the 'messy' world of practice, with nursing students being exposed to a learning strategy that encourages deep as opposed to surface learning. Implementing PBL is not easy, and does not offer a 'quick fix' (Margetson, 1997). It will present unique challenges and there will be difficulties in implementing the process of PBL, encouraging students to expand their learning repertoire and challenging lectures to become true facilitators of learning. The rewards, however, are in our opinion, worth striving for if we truly believe in developing 'lifelong learners' who will take nursing practice, research and education on to its next level of development.

References

Alavi, C (1995) Introduction, in Alavi, C (ed) *Problem-based Learning in a Health Sciences Curriculum*, London: Routledge.

Albanese, M A and Mitchell, S (1993) Problem-based learning: A review of the literature on its outcomes and implementation issues, *Academic Medicine*, **68**(1): 52–81.

Alexander, M A (1983) *Learning to Nurse: Intergrating Theory and Practice,* Edinburgh: Churchill Livingstone.

Amos, E and White, M J (1998) Teaching Tools: Problem-based learning, *Nurse Educator,* 23(2): 11–14.

Barrows, H S and Tamblyn, R M (1980) *Problem-based Learning: An Approach to Medical Education,* New York: Springer.

Bawden, R (1997) Towards a Praxis of situation improving. In Boud, D and Feletti, G (eds) *The Challenge of Problem-based Learning* (2nd edn), London: Kogan Page.

Bevis, Em O and Watson, J (1989) *Toward a Caring Curriculum: A New Pedagogy for Nursing,* New York: National League for Nursing.

Biley, F C and Smith, K (1998) 'The buck stops here': accepting responsibility for learning and actions after graduation from a problem-based learning nursing education curriculum, *Journal of Advanced Nursing,* 27: 1021–9.

Boud, D and Feletti, G (1991) Introduction. In Boud, D and Feletti, G (eds) *The Challenge of Problem-based Learning,* London: Kogan Page.

Boud, D and Feletti, G (1997) Changing Problem-based learning. Introduction to the Second Edition. In Boud, D and Feletti, G (eds) *The Challenge of Problem-based Learning* (2nd edn), London: Kogan Page.

Boud, D and Feletti, G (1997) What is Problem-based Learning? In Boud, D and Feletti, G (eds) *The Challenge of Problem-based Learning* (2nd edn), London: Kogan Page.

Cavanagh, S J and Coffin, D A (1994) Matching instructional preferences and teaching styles: A review of the literature, *Nurse Education Today,* 14: 106–10.

Cavanagh, S J, Hogan, K and Ramgopal, T (1994) Student nurse learning styles, *Senior Nurse,* 13(7): 37–41.

Coles, C (1997) Is problem-based learning the only way? In Boud, D and Feletti, G (eds) *The Challenge of Problem-based Learning* (2nd edn), London: Kogan Page.

Creedy, D and Alavi, C (1997) Problem-based learning in an integrated nursing curriculum. In Boud, D and Feletti, G (eds) *The Challenge of Problem-based Learning* (2nd edn), London: Kogan Page.

Des Marchais, J (1993) A students-centered, problem-based curriculum: 5 years' experience, *Canadian Medical Association,* 149(9): 1567–72.

Doring, A, Bramwell-Vial, A and Bingham, B (1995) Staff comfort/ discomfort with problem-based learning: A preliminary study, *Nurse Education Today,* 15(4): 263–6.

Griggs, D B and Griggs, S A (1998) Learning styles and the nursing profession. In Dunn, R and Griggs, S A (eds) *Learning Styles and the Nursing Profession,* New York: National League for Nurses.

Happell, B (1998) Problem-based learning: providing hope for psychiatric nursing? *Nurse Education Today,* 18: 362–7.

MacDonald, P J (1991) Selection of Health Problems for a problem-based Curriculum. In Boud, D and Feletti, G (eds) *The Challenge of Problem-based Learning,* London: Kogan Page.

Margetson, D (1994) Current Educational Reform and the Significance of Problem-based Learning, *Studies in Higher Education,* **19**(1): 5–19.

Margetson, D (1997) Why is Problem-based Learning a Challenge? In Boud, D and Feletti, G (eds) *The Challenge of Problem-based Learning* (2nd edn), London: Kogan Page.

Marton, F and Saljo, R (1984) Approaches to learning. In Marton, F, Hounsell, D and Entwistle, N J (eds) *The Experience of Learning,* Edinburgh: Scottish Academic Press.

McIntosh, J, Veitch, L and May, N (1997) Evaluation of Nurse and Midwife Education in Scotland, *Nursing Times,* **93**(19): 46–8.

Miller, A (1985) The relationship between nursing theory and nursing practice, *Journal of Advanced Nursing,* **10**(5): 417–24.

Partridge, S (1983) Learning styles: a review of selected models, *Journal of Nurse Education,* **22**(20): 243–8.

Ramprogus, V K (1988) Learning how to learn, *Journal of Advanced Nursing,* **8**: 59–67.

Ramsden, P (1991) *Learning to Teach In Higher Education,* London: Routledge.

Rono, F (1997) A students' review of the challenges and limitations of problem-based learning, *Education for Health,* **10**(2), 199–204.

Runciman, P, Dewar, B and Goulbourne, A (1998) *Project 2000 in Scotland: Employers' needs and the skills of newly qualified project 2000 staff nurses. Executive Summary,* Edinburgh: Queen Margaret College.

Ryan, G (1993) Student Perceptions about Self-directed Learning in a professional Programme Implementing Problem-based learning, *Studies in Higher Education,* **18**(1): 53–63.

Ryan, G and Lyttle, P (1991) Innovation in a nursing curriculum: A process of change. In Boud, D and Feletti, G (eds) *The Challenge of Problem-based Learning,* London: Kogan Page.

Sadlo, G, Waren Piper, D and Agnew, P (1994) Problem-based learning in the development of an Occupational Therapy Curriculum, Part 1: The process of problem-based learning, *British Journal of Occupational Therapy,* **57**(2): 49–54.

Savin-Baden, M (2000) *Problem-based Learning in Higher Education: Untold Stories,* Buckingham: The Society for Research into Higher Education and Open University Press.

Schwartz, R W, Burgett, J E, Blue, A V, Donnelly, M B and Sloan, D A (1997) Problem-based learning and performance-based testing: effective alternatives for undergraduate surgical education and assessment of students performance, *Medical Teacher,* **19**(10): 19–23.

Stern, P (1997) Student perceptions of a problem-based learning programme, *The American Journal of Occupational Therapy,* **51**(7): 589–96.

Townsend, J (1990) Problem-based learning, *Nursing Times,* **86**(14): 61–2.

UKCC (1999) *Fitness for Practice: The UKCC Commission for Nursing and Midwifery Education,* London: UKCC.

Vaughan, J A (1990) Student nurse attitudes to teaching/learning methods, *Journal of Advanced Nursing,* **15**: 925–33.

WHO (1993) *Increasing the relevance of education for health professionals: A report of a WHO study group on problem-solving education for the health professions,* Geneva: WHO.

Williams, L (1998) Study Matters, *Nursing Times,* **12**(36): 4.

3

Creating The Problem

Introduction

This chapter considers the nature of problems, their construction, presentation and evaluation. It aims to help you to understand how to develop material for use in PBL sessions. As discussed in Chapter 1, the term 'problem' is in itself problematical. In this chapter the term 'problem' is used to refer to the actual material used to stimulate student learning. The problem has two components; a 'trigger' which 'triggers' the PBL process and creates the stimulus for learning and a description of the situation in which the student is expected to deal with the problem, usually in the role of a registered nurse. The trigger and the situation combined are sometimes referred to as the 'scenario' or the 'case' (case-based learning is different from, although similar to, problem-based learning), the situation improvement package (SIP) or the situation in need of improvement (SINI).

In this chapter the trigger material plus the description of the situation will be referred to as the 'scenario'. To create a 'PBL package' a guide for the facilitator is added to the trigger and situation. The facilitator guide contains further information about the topic to be studied, including the expected learning outcomes, along with material such as prompt questions and detail of resources such as relevant lectures, workshops, and laboratory sessions. The package may also contain references, web sites and names and telephone numbers of experts who are willing to be contacted by students. Additional information about the patient or client in the scenario may also be included, for example blood results or home circumstances, as may material related to any diagnostic procedures undertaken or nursing assessments made. Packages can vary in size from a single page to in excess of

50 pages. The amount of material in each package will depend on the complexity of the topic, the level of the students and the amount of time allocated to the package. Most PBL packages run over at least three sessions interspersed with time for self-study: an introductory session where the trigger is presented and discussion takes place and learning needs are identified; one or more review sessions (which may or may not be facilitated), where issues can be redefined and information exchanged and a feedback session where learning is integrated to suggest and justify nursing interventions which would produce an improvement in the described situation.

Material for use in PBL can be obtained from other institutions or from commercial organisations that supply either the trigger material alone or the trigger material and suggested facilitator questions. Wade (1999) stated that as the time and resources needed to develop valid scenarios are not often available, commercially produced material could be useful. However, one of the strengths of PBL as a learning strategy is that it is contextualised and thus reflects local situations and environments. PBL is flexible and, unlike purchased material, can be readily adapted to suit the needs of individual programmes and to reflect the rapid and frequent changes in the provision and delivery of health care. For these reasons it is almost always better for individual institutions to develop their own PBL material to suit their own programmes.

The nature of the scenario

Scenarios are central to the PBL process. They can serve a variety of purposes. Primarily, they provide a basis for discussion in a non-threatening environment. They can be used to illustrate and apply theoretical concepts to the practice situation in an integrated manner. Collaborative working and interpersonal skills, including toleration and respect for others' beliefs, can be developed. Analysis of the scenarios stimulates thought with the need to justify one's response assisting in the development of critical thinking while promoting evidence-based practice. The ability of PBL to develop these lifelong learning skills is sometimes referred to as the 'value added' by PBL.

A good scenario brings reality into the classroom and forces students to put themselves in the role of decision-maker and problem-solver. Not only do students gain the appropriate propositional knowledge needed to provide nursing care for the client in the scenario, the dissecting and reconstructing of the situation promotes examination of personal value systems and an understanding of themselves and others in the team (Wade, 1999).

Duch (1996) identified characteristics of 'good' PBL scenarios. She stated that problems must attract the students' interest and motivate them to seek further information about the issues involved. Thus an important feature of a PBL scenario is that it reflects reality. The situation needs to 'smell real' to the student and stimulate the required learning. Students need to feel that the situation is indeed one in which they are likely to find themselves in practice settings. Scenarios therefore should be drawn from recent relevant clinical experience. It is helpful to have a member or members of clinical staff on the scenario writing team. Preceptors or mentors are excellent sources of situations that can be adapted to create PBL scenarios. If real life situations are used directly it is essential to ensure that patient permission is sought and that confidentiality is maintained. In ensuring this, scenario writers may alter details or combine aspects from two or more patient cases. Where a combination of cases is used, scenario writers must take care that the 'smell real' factor is maintained and that the 'patient with everything' is not presented in one scenario. Students quickly develop the skill to distinguish 'made up' patients from the genuine article. Learning in context is a major strength of PBL but the context has to be genuine.

Students can also provide their own scenarios. In addition to using PBL in theoretical modules, the Hogheschule Limburg in The Netherlands operates a system called 'out school PBL' (Heijen, 1997). Students are encouraged to utilise the PBL process when reflecting on their practice placements. On return days in school, students describe practice situations about which they feel they require more learning. The PBL group decides which of the situations to explore further and proceeds to identify learning needs. Good problems require students to make decisions or judgements based on facts, information, logic and/or rationalisation. The problems presented must have a solvable solution. This does not imply that the scenario has to present a simple, clear-cut case that has a single 'right answer'. Many situations encountered in nursing are untidy and do not have a single correct intervention, so-called 'messy problems'. These types of problems are ideal for PBL as they provide the opportunity for students to discuss the issues involved (Sadlo, 1995). The open-ended nature of the 'solution' challenges students to reason and to argue their case, rather than each student selecting an issue to present. Inclusion of controversial scenarios keeps students functioning as a team, drawing on each other's knowledge and integrating knowledge. It should be possible to suggest solutions or at least improve most scenarios. There is little point in presenting students with scenarios that depict the worst possible case in which little could be done to at least resolve the situation (Wade, 1999).

PBL promotes evidence-based practice by requiring students to justify their selected nursing interventions through the use of up-to-date research material. The evidence on which students base their decisions should be readily available. Just as the situations to be explored should be encountered frequently in practice, there is equally little gain in presenting students with problems about which there is little published research-based evidence. The unimagined increase in information technology since the development of PBL in the 1960s has improved ease of access to the evidence. In particular use of the World Wide Web will supply information on almost any topic. The problem facing present day facilitators may not be students' inability to find supporting evidence, but their ability to judge the quality of articles which range from personal opinion to the results of rigorous research.

The description of the problem should be neutral and focus on an aspect that requires further exploration. It should be concrete, not contain too many distractions and limit the number of issues that can be identified. Hafler (1997) in a study of PBL case writers found that there was a risk of including too many irrelevant details. The more detail that is given, the more distractions arise to divert students from the main issues to be explored. While the inclusion of 'red herrings' may be used intentionally with final year students to develop prioritisation skills, too much information can confuse new students. An example from the authors' experience involved a community nursing scenario concerning an elderly gentleman with depression and weight loss that mentioned a septic tank (a waste collection unit used for isolated premises not connected to main sewerage). This had been included to indicate that the client's house was situated in a remote part of the country.

Students were unfamiliar with the arrangement and spent a great deal of time exploring septic tanks, their design, installation and emptying at the expense of the intended issue of providing community nursing services to people in isolated rural areas. The authors' experience indicates that for pre-registration nursing students small scenarios work best. Students have to consider a broad range of options rather than concentrating on a highly specific case. As information about clients, in reality, is often incomplete, students need to develop skills to work with the facts available and to be able identify what further information is really necessary. Jones and Sheridan (1999) claimed that good scenarios are 'small segments of reality'; clear, concise fact-filled cases that promote discussion.

Creating a PBL scenario

Although PBL can be implemented as a philosophy which permeates the entire curriculum, in nurse education it is primarily a learning/teaching strategy. PBL packages must be matched to the desired outcomes of the programme in which they are used. Thus the first step in developing PBL packages must be integrated with curriculum development. The learning outcomes, programme content and practice experience form the basis for the focus of the PBL triggers and guide the order in which they will occur. The programme structure, modules, terms and themes will inform the focus of the PBL packages, the number of packages in any term and the time allocated to each package and individual PBL session. Alavi (1995), suggested the use of grids to map the content of PBL scenarios against learning outcomes (Figure 3.1) to ensure that all material is contained within the PBL scenarios for any given module. The flow-through of content and themes that progress from one module to another should also be considered in relation to the PBL packages at this stage.

In programmes where PBL is not the sole learning strategy, the order of PBL packages will usually reflect the increasing academic level. Academic level may be of lesser importance when considering the content of PBL packages. Barrows (1988) stated that most first year students have some conception of human biology and caring needs and thus can be exposed to patient problems from

DIPLOMA OF HIGHER EDUCATION IN NURSING
FOUNDATION PROGRAMME
MODULE ONE

PBL Scenarios

Module Topics	The Book's Thing	Images of Ourselves	Admitting Doris	Mrs Blair's Holiday	First Cut is the Deepest	Mr Dougal Goes Home
Literature search	●	●	●	●	●	●
Referencing technique	●	●				
Professional issues		●	●			●
Admission procedure			●			
Patient assessment			●	●	●	●
Communication			●	●	●	●
Hygiene skills				●	●	
Continence promotion				●		●
Nutrition			●	●	●	●
Infection control				●	●	
Patient observation			●	●	●	●
Fluid balance				●	●	
Moving and handling				●	●	●
Multi-disciplinary team				●	●	●
Discharge planning			●		●	●

Figure 3.1   Scenario: topic grid

the beginning stages of a programme. This view is supported by Margetson (1994) who argued that PBL required a coherentist view of learning, in which knowledge is part of living and is acquired for its own sake not for passing tests, rather than a foundationalist perception of learning which requires that 'foundation' knowledge must be acquired before more complex issues can be addressed. The latter view is sometimes compared to building blocks where 'higher' blocks cannot be placed until the lower blocks or foundation are in place, whereas in the coherentist view, knowledge can be compared to an onion, the layers of which can be peeled back one or more at a time, either in complete layers or in parts of layers. If this argument is accepted, PBL packages can involve material of any complexity at any point in the programme, as students will learn to the level that is required to find a solution to the problem.

In practice PBL packages tend to be developed for specific points within programmes. Duch (1996) recommends the use of a taxonomy such as that of Bloom (1956) to assist in the ordering of scenarios. Although the expected level of the scenarios may be geared to academic levels, students can begin decision-making from the first year. Students can also explore issues beyond the depth required for the academic level. The material to be learned through a problem-based approach should be integrated rather than subject-based. It may reflect or be supported by other learning strategies used in the programme, but should not replicate content learned by other methods. While some programmes are designed as 'pure' PBL, i.e. PBL scenarios are the only learning/teaching strategy used, most problem-based nursing programmes employ other teaching methodologies, such as lectures, open learning material, laboratory work and, in particular, clinical skills sessions. It is helpful if the programme timetable is temporally co-ordinated to ensure that different topic areas, such as life or social sciences, complement each other and support the central focus of nursing. Thus a PBL scenario focussing on the assessment of a client might be timetabled to co-ordinate with workshops on the use of nursing assessment tools, clinical skills sessions on patient observation and interviewing, lectures on communication theories and the physiology of blood pressure, temperature and pulse. It is important that lecturers are aware of the content of sessions other than their own and that subjects are not over-taught. PBL aims to give students control over their own learning. Too many supporting lectures can defeat this purpose. Students quickly lose the motivation for self-directed learning if they feel that all the answers are provided in lectures. PBL is acknowledged as a teacher-intensive strategy. Few institutions have the resources to facilitate PBL in addition to undertaking unnecessary teaching in fixed resources.

Providing the context

The curriculum document will indicate the content, level and order of the PBL scenarios but it does not provide the detail of the patient/client, the context of the situation or the value to be added through the use of PBL. Content may be focused on topics such as disorders or disabilities, nursing activities, professional issues, and health promotion. The scenarios should reflect an environment in which the student is likely to be placed, for example acute wards, intensive care units, nursing homes, patients' homes, prisons. The situation may also require the student to adopt one specific nursing role such as health educator, care provider, resource manager rather than only stating 'registered nurse'.

There is debate as to whether or not students should be asked to consider roles that they are unlikely to encounter in their initial programme. Although the purchasing of nurse education by either NHS Trust confederation in England and Wales or the Scottish and Northern Irish Executives, is based on local requirements, there is no guarantee that nurses will remain in the geographical area in which they originally trained. It can therefore be argued that it is acceptable to ask students to consider roles such as those of specialist practitioners that they may encounter in other NHS Trusts or in the independent sector.

The patient conditions and caring environments chosen should reflect situations that the students are likely to encounter. In the UK, adult nursing students will certainly care for patients with cardiovascular disease and mental health students for clients with dementia. Treatment care plans should be evidence-based. Thus there will be some similarity between plans produced in London and Wick, but there will be local differences in terms of available resources, implementation policies and guidelines. These 'post-code' differences will be reflected in the students' response to the trigger.

Scenarios should be diverse and reflect the range of situations likely to be encountered by students. The challenge of considering different scenarios, presented in different formats, helps to develop critical thinking skills and also to prevent student boredom (Alavi, 1995; Jones and Sheridan, 1999).

In addition to the content, consideration should be given to the 'value-added' elements of PBL. These may promote skills such as team working, presentation of case or critical thinking. Students can be required to apply analytical tools, prioritise data, articulate issues within the scenario or reflect on experience. As the experience and knowledge base of the students' increases, they will be expected to draw on previous knowledge, making links, integrating and applying it to new situations. Students working through a problem-based programme acquire substantive knowledge, develop analytical and team working skills and gain in self-confidence (Boehrer and Linskey, 1990). These skills form the basis for lifelong learning, a necessary requirement in the rapidly developing and ever-changing climate of professional nursing practice.

Activity 3.1

Think of a topic such as a client group, a condition, a professional issue, a treatment or a skill about which either you or your students need to learn more.

Narrow the topic to three or four issues and write outcomes for the learning you expect to be achieved.

Creating the scenario

When the decisions about focus and content have been made, the production of PBL scenarios passes to the writing team. Ideally, PBL scenarios should be written by a team that develops increasing expertise in the art of scenario creation. As scenario writing is a time consuming activity, it has been suggested that the writing team be freed up from other activities (Hengstberger-Sims and McMillan, 1993). While this has the attraction of allowing work to proceed unimpeded, it has some drawbacks. Few Schools of Nursing have sufficient staff to release three or more members from teaching activities completely. Loss of staff from the writing team through retirement, promotion and movement may lead to difficulties at a later date. A small number of writers may have insufficient expertise to contribute to all content areas. The Staff who create the PBL packages need to have an awareness of all parts of the programme to ensure that the PBL scenario matches the level of the programme, triggers appropriate learning and is adequately resourced. All of these are easier to achieve if teachers are actively involved in delivering the programme. Hafler (1997) reported that scenario writers found scenarios easier to write when they were involved in teaching the subject. While there is considerable debate as to whether or not PBL facilitators need to be topic experts or if sound facilitation skills are preferable (see Chapter 6), it is essential that the people producing the package have expertise in the focus of the scenario. While most nurse teachers would be comfortable facilitating pre-registration students in branch-specific topics, they would not necessarily possess the in-depth knowledge and skills required to devise the PBL package. For post-registration programmes, topic expertise is desirable for both package creation and facilitation.

As it is unlikely that a writing team of three or four teachers will possess all the expertise needed to create all of the scenarios in a programme, an alternative method is to have several teams undertaking the writing of scenarios. Co-ordination across teams is essential if this approach is adopted to ensure that triggers are not repetitive and that all scenarios are equal in complexity and time required for completion for any given point in the programme. The inclusion of clinical staff in writing teams helps to keep the reality of the trigger and ensures that material in the facilitator guide reflects the local practice that will be experienced by students. Clinical staff time for educational purposes may be restricted so flexibility and innovation is required. Silver *et al.* (1999) described a project where teachers from different disciplines and different sites worked together to create six PBL scenarios related to care of the older adult. A primary team of three or four people produced the learning objectives, cases and specific guidelines. This material was subsequently reviewed by a different team and a final edit carried out by the whole team.

Silver *et al.* (1999) stated that the project had increased awareness of other disciplines, an attribute that they hoped the students would mirror in working through the PBL material, and had improved faculty staff familiarity with the PBL process. Several difficulties were also identified. Scheduling of other commitments made working difficult, especially as staff were based on different sites and the distance between sites led to travelling difficulties. Other methods of working were tried, including use of an Internet chat room. It was felt that loss of face-to-face interaction led to a reduction in dynamism and enthusiasm. The authors have had a similar experience using video conferencing and agree that even this visual method detracts from the creative process.

PBL is resource intensive, making particularly heavy demands not only on journals, books, Internet access and computerised data bases but also on library staff. Inclusion of librarians at some point in the creative phase is essential. Clinical experts who may not be available to participate in the writing can act as a valuable contact for students. Individuals and agencies that may be willing to act as specialised resources should also be approached for permission as part of the scenario development.

Activity 3.2

Using the topic and outcomes from the first activity, think about other people who might be helpful in developing a scenario based on your chosen topic. They might be subject experts such as your preceptor/mentor, staff in your link area, friends with a different perspective on life or your personal teacher. You may want to work with them in developing a scenario or you may want to ask them to review the finished package.

Now make a list of people and/or organisations that might be willing to provide expert advice on the subject.

Triggers

The layout of a situation and the associated facilitators' guides often follow a house style. It is in the development of the triggers that creativity can be given free rein. Video, cartoon, poem, photograph – the range of material that can be used as a trigger for learning is bounded only by the writer's imagination.

Paper cases

Cases are often described as the patient's story. They are frequently referred to as an inseparable part of PBL, although it is possible to utilise cases as a problem-solving learning strategy without adopting all of the characteristics of PBL. It can be argued that all triggers, however presented, represent a case to a greater or lesser degree. Cases are traditionally presented in a paper format. Several institutions use paper cases to the exclusion of all other trigger forms. The patient information contained in the trigger may be brief, two or three lines, or fairly extensive, the size of a set of full case notes. The amount and type of information in the cases varies from minimal patient biographical detail to complete nursing and medical assessment, including the results of diagnostic tests. The amount of detail given should relate to the issues to be triggered – there is little point in providing the information that the client lives in a two-bedroomed flat if the student is not required to utilise this information in identifying issues from the scenario. In some forms of paper cases more information is available, but students have to ask specific questions and justify to the facilitator why they need to know that detail in order to be given the information. Experience will tell if this is a suitable strategy for a particular programme or not. Sometimes students find a lack of detail frustrating, at other times the amount of detail available confuses the issue. Cases may be presented as unfolding over a time scale. Students identify issues, return with the new knowledge and are then given more details about the patient. Patients can be revisited at different points in their history and at different points in the programme. Care should be taken when using the same clients as over-use of particular clients can lead to student boredom and feelings of *deja-vu*.

Building of scenarios

When the desired learning outcomes and the focus of the PBL session have been decided, scenarios can be built up in a variety of ways, as in the following example.

Example

Trigger
Mrs Laura Fouchetti, a 42-year-old mother of four, has just returned to the ward following a laproscopic cholecystectomy.

The situation is now added. This should reflect the knowledge and experience of the student. Pre-registration students are usually expected to take the role of D grade staff nurses.

As her named nurse ....

An indication of what learning is required can be given by indicating an action pertinent to the scenario

..................you have to plan Mrs Fouchetti's nursing care requirement for the next 48 hours.

A prompt of this type is useful when designing scenarios for junior students. If the scenario is intended for qualified staff, you may want to omit the learning prompt and leave the situation completely open.

A brief scenario of the sort exemplified above type should prompt questions related to:

- the reasons for cholecystectomy, including the anatomy and physiology of the gall bladder and the aetiology and pathology of gall stones
- differences between laproscopic and open surgery
- the patient's likely status on the return to the ward for example, intravenous infusion, drains etc
- potential complications and how to prevent them
- pre-discharge advice

The scenario could also be triggered by using charts such as a post-operative recovery form or a transcript of the recovery room nurse's handover to the ward nurse.

The trigger can be adapted to shift the focus of the learning or to increase the complexity of the situation.

For example – by adding another sentence to the initial trigger
She asks you 'Did they find anything nasty?'
will trigger learning related to:

- patient/nurse communication
- patient education
- reassurance
- breaking bad news

Despite having patient-controlled analgesia (PCA) in situ she complains of pain
will stimulate learning related to:

- pain-controlled analgesia, mechanisms, effectiveness, substances used

– physiology/psychology of pain
– possible causes of post-operative pain
– alternative/complementary methods of pain relief including
  legislation governing their use by nurses

Alterations can also be made to the situation and intervention

............*begin discharge planning*

............*explain to a first year student nurse what procedure has been undertaken/why this nursing care is required*

The scenario can be extended to add issues such as hospital-acquired infection, deep venous thrombosis, anxiety over body image and so on. Likewise the amount of information given could be expanded to include admission assessment sheets, theatre checklists, fluid balance charts and so forth. The temptation to pad out the trigger with detail can be attractive to novice scenario writers as it may be difficult to believe that a three or four line trigger will encourage students to achieve the necessary learning. Students are often surprised at the amount they learn from short scenarios and often identify pertinent issues that are at a more complex level that required by the scenario.

Paper cases can be used to trigger learning about specific aspects of nursing care. Jordan (1996) described the use of paper cases in the learning of pharmacology. Cases were used to provide narratives that illustrated difficult aspects of therapeutic treatment and assisted in linking pharmacological theory with practice. Jordan found that the cases, although focusing on pharmacology, triggered discussion of other areas such as nursing ethics. Narratives supplied by students provided powerful cases for future classes. Care is required to ensure that the cases do not become too blurred and present an overload of information.

Video or audio-tapes

Video clips can also be used as triggers. As these often have considerable impact their effect can be very powerful. Students can add their own observations, for example, of facial expression, voice tone, skin appearance, body build and personal appearance, to the information given on the clip and to the situation. Video clips can be taken from commercially supplied videos or can be custom-made by the institution. Commercially supplied videos are expensive (multiple copies may be required), tend to date quickly and may not fully meet the needs of the scenario. The impact of the clip must be weighed against the cost of buying or renting several copies of the whole video for the sake of a 5-minute segment. It is temping to 'bootleg' copies of emotive television productions, but penalties for illegal screening are high and seeking permission may lead to copyright problems for multiple copies or multiple viewings. In-house recordings are free of copyright problems, can be scripted to reflect the local context and can be adapted as required. The improvements in the quality of audio-visual equipment available in most institutions makes this a feasible option, although script writing, filming and making multiple copies is a time consuming process. We suggest that non-teaching staff such as simulated patients or willing family or friends, are used in the video as students may have difficulty in accepting known staff in patient roles. Videos can also be made in the clinical area with the proviso that patient informed consent is obtained and confidentiality is ensured. Such triggers have the advantage of 'feeling very real' and are readily identified with by students.

Audio-tapes can also provide trigger material. While the impact is less than that of video-tape, students have to listen carefully to notice the information from the tape and the nuances of voice tone, word emphasis and pauses.

Simulated patients

Simulated patients are a valued resource used increasingly in many institutions that educate health care professionals. Simulated patients may be volunteers or paid actors but all are trained to take the role of one or more patients with specific disorders. For nursing programmes, the patient role may include socio-economic or psychological issues as well as physical symptoms. Simulated patients may also enact the part of relatives or carers. In a PBL setting, simulated patients provide the trigger. Students have a limited time in which to interview or assess the simulated patient in order to determine the issues. This provides 'value-added' issues related to interviewing, especially in asking the right questions and acting on patient responses – verbal and non-verbal. Feedback from simulated patients to students can be very valuable as it often carries more impact than the same comment given by the facilitator. Preparation of simulated patients is all-important. Simulated patients must be adequately informed of what the scenario is about and what the students are expected to gain from it. Real patients can also act as 'triggers'. VanLeit (1995) described a project which involved real patients participating in an occupational therapy programme where clients who had had input from occupational therapists agreed to meet with occupational therapy (OT) students. Contact with real clients encouraged students to explore the theoretical underpinnings of OT interventions and to relate them to the pragmatics of the situation and the patients' experience. Aspegren, Blomquist and Borgstrom (1998) reported on the involvement of real patients in an undergraduate medical curriculum. Students, in their PBL teams, examined and interviewed patients in a surgical outpatient clinic. Following the contact with the patient, the students met with a facilitator to identify the issues associated with the patient and then worked through the PBL process. When asked to compare paper cases with real patients, none of the students preferred paper cases alone. None of the patients felt distressed by participating in the PBL session and several commented that it had been enjoyable. Aspegren *et al.* (1998) stressed that patients must be carefully chosen and must give informed consent. Given the large numbers of patients who would be required to support nursing programmes, use of real patients may not be an option for problem-based programmes in nursing.

Poetry and literature

Short extracts from literature or poems can be used to trigger learning. Most nurses are familiar with the poem about the old lady asking nurses what they see when they look at her. This can be used to stimulate learning about ageing and ageism. Writings by patients describing experience can also generate issues to be explored further. Articles or headlines from papers can be used to introduce controversial or highly topical issues. One PBL session in a programme can be left 'blank' for a topical issue that can be decided and added at very short notice, ensuring that the programme is always up to date.

Pictures

Pictures may be classical art, photographs, cartoons or from the media. Famous paintings can be used to introduce the nature of caring or recruitment posters to trigger learning about nursing history. A series of photographs can be used to show changes in a person over time to trigger learning about, for example, dementia, multiple sclerosis, the results of brain damage and the feelings and needs of relatives, especially if they are lay carers. Cartoons may provide a short story that raises issues or a situation that needs to be resolved.

Pieces of equipment

Items of equipment also make good triggers. For example a dialyser from a haemodialysis machine will trigger issues related to what is it? how does it work?, why would you need it? From these questions should come learning about renal physiology, chronic renal failure and associated nursing interventions.

Music

Music can be used to trigger learning. Many songs reflect a comment on society or a state of mind or tell a story that can be linked to, for example, the effect of environment on health or caring for clients with mental health problems.

Computer-based triggers

Computers are being increasingly used in PBL, not only as a resource but also as triggers. Cheek, Gillham and Mills (1997) described the integration of a computerised clinical database with PBL scenarios on Acute Care Nursing. The scenarios encouraged reflective thinking around a variety of practical problems, simulated patient progress and documentation. Students were asked to compile care plans around the scenarios using the database. In addition to promoting the PBL objectives of promoting teamwork, encouraging collaboration, encouraging reflective practice, promoting respect and encouraging continuous improvement, the computing component of the module was integrated with nursing content in a context in which it would be used by students in placements.

Computer-based learning is usually regarded as an individual experience, whereas the PBL philosophy stresses group interaction and teamwork. However PBL has been used successfully in open and distance learning by individual students (Price, 2000).

Computers can also be used interactively to simulate patients. White (1995) described the use of interactive video added to computer programmes. This had the advantage of allowing students to interact with the patient on the video allowing the result of interventions to be seen. Advances in computing and artificial intelligence have taken this further. Students can interview and examine patients in a more meaningful way. Albion and Gibson (1998) described the application of PBL principles with Interactive Multimedia (IMM). The project was designed to stimulate processes similar to the PBL processes. Students have access to sample responses prepared by a group after they have completed the tasks. Advances in Artificial Intelligence may make it possible for the computer to provide the role of facilitator in the future.

Although many institutions now provide student access to both Internet and Intranet, resources are not infinite. Use of computer-based triggers or resources will place demands on expensive resources. It will also require facilitators to be sufficiently computer-literate to assist students who may not be well orientated towards computers.

Activity 3.3

Go back to the topic you identified in the previous activity. Think about two or three ways in which you could present a trigger that would stimulate people to learn more about the topic. Now write a situation to go with one trigger.

Ask a colleague or colleagues to 'brainstorm' each of the triggers and write down all the issues that come into their minds.

Compare their list with the outcomes you developed.

Which trigger produced the closest match with the outcomes you identified? How could you trigger the missing issues?

Do your colleagues know everything about the issues that they identified or would they need to find out more?

How could you prompt learning about the issues that have been missed?

Facilitator's guide

The facilitator's guide should be produced in tandem with the scenario, by the same writing team. As discussed earlier there has been some debate around the attributes required by a PBL facilitator. These will be discussed further in Chapters 4 and 5. The facilitator's guide should contain sufficient material to assist facilitators to help students towards the intended learning and to provide guidance on the material that they should expect to be produced at the feedback sessions. While it can be argued that good facilitation skills can compensate for lack of in-depth specialist knowledge at pre-registration level, the facilitator guides, like the scenarios, should be written by people with up-to-date, in-depth knowledge of the topic area. Annual review dates should be set to up-date the information and to review the overall effectiveness of the scenario.

Learning outcomes

Facilitator's guides should contain the outcomes expected for the session. Should the outcomes be given to students in advance, with the scenario, after the feedback or not at all? On the one hand, PBL is claimed to be highly student-centred with students having control over learning – why should learning outcomes be dictated by the Institution? On the other, nursing and midwifery programmes have to produce practitioners who are 'fit for purpose'. Competencies must be achieved for registration to be awarded. Schools must have proof that they are teaching to the validated programme documents, which state the outcomes. If students can pick and choose their own learning outcomes, how can the school be sure that they will achieve the outcomes? PBL scenarios should be constructed to ensure that students will identify appropriate learning outcomes, without being too restrictive or constraining. The facilitator's guide should contain learning outcomes. Whether or not these are issued to students prior to/with the scenario is a matter for discussion by the programme planning team.

Our experience has been that giving learning outcomes for each PBL session to students, limits the discussion. Students quickly identify what is expected and, being students, divide up the content to be examined. They end up knowing only the part of the topic they studied. The knowledge gained from discussion and challenge is missing. The overall learning outcomes for the term or module are usually available to students in module/programme handbooks. Students can then check their PBL outcomes against the outcomes after each module. It is possible to allow students to select which PBL scenario they want to undertake in order to meet the remaining learning outcomes. This strategy depends on the availability of a range of PBL packages and an open approach to fixed resources. In addition to the outcomes related to student learning, the guide should also contain outcomes related to the PBL process and the facilitator's role in achieving the expectations of the scenario.

Example

In the example of Mrs Fouchetti the learning outcomes for the students might be:

1. Describe the structure and function of the gall bladder
2. Explain the formation of gallstones
3. Outline the medical treatment of gallstones
4. Plan post-operative care for a patient following cholecystectomy, giving rationales for your actions
5. Identify the advice that would be given to a patient before discharge following cholecystectomy. Give reasons for your choices.

And for the facilitator:

1. Promote discussion and identification of issues related to the PBL scenario
2. Assist the PBL team to clarify their learning needs
3. Encourage collaborative working
4. Assist the team to identify potential learning resources
5. Encourage discussion and challenge among team members.

Content
An outline of the expected content should be provided. This may be divided into knowledge, skills and attitude components.

The **knowledge** component should reflect the programme content for the module, which in turn should be appropriate to the level of the student, matching prior learning and material yet to come.

Activity 3.4
Identify the content you expect students to obtain in response to the situation developed in the previous activities.

The **skills** component should reflect the so-called nursing or clinical skills such as bathing, oral hygiene, aseptic technique, PEG feeding, pain assessment and information giving. These should be linked to the underpinning evidence in the feedback session. They may or may not be demonstrated (see Chapter 8 for feedback) within the PBL session. The selected 'value added' aspects of PBL such as team-working, questioning and critical thinking may be included in this section.

Activity 3.5
List the clinical skills that you think nurses need to improve the situation you have developed. Remember to include skills linked to assessment and communication in addition to psychomotor skills.

What value do you expect PBL to add the students learning e.g. rationale for actions, ability to think things through logically?

The **attitude** component should indicate the stance you expect students to take towards the situation. It should reflect ethical judgements and a caring ethos. You should expect this component to be demonstrated in the PBL sessions, students should speak of patients/clients with respect and adopt a non-judgemental attitude.

Activity 3.6
Identify the attitude component that you would expect to be adopted by registered nurses in the situation you have described.

In addition to outcomes and content it is often useful to include an overview of the timing of the sessions. Obviously as these are student-led, the timings may vary considerably – however facilitators have indicated that it is useful to have some idea about the material to be covered to assist students in moving the discussion along. As PBL sessions may be spread over a variable number of sessions, it is helpful to have an overview of this at the start of each session. Although PBL is student-centred and the issues are generated by students, facilitators report that it is useful to have one or two 'prompt' questions in the package for those occasions when discussion comes to a halt and no-one is sure what to do next (see Chapter 7 on managing dysfunction and disjunction).

Problem-based learning packages may also contain reference lists and lists of other resources. Students rapidly learn to search the timetables for lectures on related material. It should be stressed that PBL sessions are not a re-presentation of lecture/ workshop content but should include new material from published sources. Useful web sites can also be included along with names and contact information for experts (either within or outside the institution), who have agreed to talk to students. Only one or two people from each PBL group should approach experts to avoid overload.

Package preview sessions should be held prior to the introduction of new PBL scenarios into the programme. The preview sessions give the writing team the opportunity to describe the package to the other facilitators and to make one or two suggestions on how they see it being used, e.g. timing of video clip; situation given before/after trigger; any extra material to be given out or only if requested by students. Facilitators can offer feedback on elements such as the package; clarity of information in situations; match with point in programme, level of student, other content, practice experience. Preferably the preview should be held sufficiently before the session to allow any necessary amendments to be made.

Evaluation of PBL packages

Packages should be reviewed after use, preferably by the facilitators and students who used them. Evaluation by students may be carried out formally by use of a questionnaire which asks about fixed attributes of the session such as clarity of the information, the degree to which the trigger stimulated learning, ease of finding supporting evidence, relevance to practice, links with other elements in the programme, perceived relevance of the topic or informally by asking student opinion. Both methods have advantages. Formal evaluation permits continuing comparison of the scenarios in use. Informal evaluation may produce issues that have been overlooked by the writing team. Facilitators' opinions regarding the running of the sessions should also be sought. Unless there is unanimous agreement on failings in scenarios, two run-throughs are recommended before changes are made in order to avoid knee-jerk responses caused by lack of familiarity on the first run-through. Open discussion helps to produce suggestions for change and also acts as a support for facilitators. Information that should be included in facilitators' guides can also be raised.

Outcomes actually obtained in sessions can be matched with the expected outcomes to assess whether the triggers are, in fact, stimulating the required learning. The outcomes can be mapped against the module/term outcomes to ensure that all are being met. Any area that is consistently ignored by students will necessitate a change to a trigger or triggers to include this area in the future. Dolmans *et al.* (1994) found that, on average, 64% of the expected outcomes were raised in the PBL trigger. Mpofu *et al.* (1997) reported a range of 55–100%, although no objective was completely omitted by the students. They suggested that the variation could result from a variety of reasons ranging from students' lack of familiarity with the PBL process to facilitator inexperience with both PBL and the local culture.

Conclusion

The creation of PBL packages requires an in-depth, up-to-date knowledge of the topic area. The integrative nature of PBL may mean that experts from two or three areas are involved, e.g. nursing skills, biological sciences and ethics. Clinical staff should be included whenever possible. Packages take time to develop and may require several rewrites to perfect. Generally package creation is an enjoyable experience, with the triggers being limited only by the creativity of the writers.

References

Alavi, C, ed (1995) *Problem-based Learning in a Health Sciences Curriculum,* Routledge: London.

Albion, P R and Gibson, I W (1998) Designing Multimedia Materials using a Problem-based Learning Design. *http://www.usq.edu.au/albion/papers/ascilite98.html*

Aspegren, K, Blomquist, P and Borgstrom, A (1998) Live patients and problem-based learning, *Medical Teacher*, **20**(5): 417–20.

Barrows, H S (1988) *The Tutorial Process*. Southern Illinois University School of Medicine: Springfield Illinois.

Bloom, B S (ed) (1956) *A Taxonomy of Educational Objectives*, Longmans, Green.

Boehrer, J and Linskey, M (1990) Teaching with Cases: Learning to Question, *New Directions for Teaching and Learning*, no **42**, summer 1990, 41–57.

Cheek, J C, Gillham, D and Mills, P (1997) Using a computerised clinical database to enhance problem-based learning strategies for second year undergraduate nursing students, *Australian Electronic Journal of Nursing Education*, **2**: 2.

Dolmans, D H J M, Wolfhagen, I A P, Schmidt, H G and van der Vleuten, C P M (1994) A rating scale for tutor evaluation in a problem-based curriculum: validity and reliability, *Medical Education*, **28**: 550–558.

Duch, B (1996) Problems: A Key Factor in PBL. *http://www.physics.udel.edu/-pbl/cte/spr96-phys*

Hafler, J P (1997) Case writing: case writers' perspectives *in* Boud, D, Feletti, G (eds) *The Challenge of Problem-based Learning*, 2nd Ed London, Kogan Page.

Heijen, R (1997) The In-School and Out-School Process According to PBL *Paper, Changing to PBL, Conference*, Brunel University September 1997.

Hengstberger-Sims, C and McMillan, M A (1993) Problem-based learning packages: considerations for neophyte package writers, *Nurse Education Today*, **13**: 73–7.

Jones, D C and Sheridan, M E (1999) A Case Study Approach: Developing Critical Thinking Skills in Novice Paediatric Nurses, *The Journal of Continuing Education in Nursing*, **30**(2): 75–8.

Jordan, S (1996) Teaching pharmacology by case study, *Nurse Education Today*, **17**(5): 386–93.

Margetson, D (1994) Current Educational Reform and the Significance of Problem-based Learning, *Studies in Higher Education*, **19**(1): 5–19.

Mpofu, D J S, Das, M, Murdoch, J C and Lanphear, J H (1997) Effectiveness of problems used in problem-based learning, *Medical Education*, **31**: 330–4

Price, B (2000) *Introducing Problem-based Learning into Distance Learning* in Glen, S and Wilkie, K (eds) (2000) *Implementing Problem-based Learning in Nursing*, Macmillan – now Palgrave Macmillan: Basingstoke.

Sadlo, G (1995) Problem-Based Learning, *Tertiary Education News*, **5**(6): 8–10.

Silver, S, Turley, M, Smith, C, Laird, J, Majewski, T, Maguire, B, Orndorff, J, Rice, L and Vowels, R (1999) Multidisciplinary Team Dynamics in the Production of Problem-Based Learning Cases in Issues Related to Older Adults, *Journal of Allied Health,* **28**(1): 21–5.

VanLeit, B (1995) Using the Case Method to Develop Clinical Reasoning Skills in Problem-Based Learning, *The American Journal of Occupational Therapy,* **49**(4): 349–53.

Wade, D (1999) Using the Case Method to Develop Critical Thinking Skills for the Care of High-Risk Families, *Journal of Family Nursing,* **5**(1): 92–109.

White, J (1995) Using Interactive Video to Add Physical Assessment Data to Computer-Based Patient Simulations in Nursing, *Computers in Nursing,* **13**(5): 233–5.

4

Introducing PBL into the Curriculum: Key Issues to Consider

Introduction

This chapter will discuss the key issues which need to be considered when introducing PBL into the curriculum. Once this decision has been made, the success or otherwise of this major educational change will depend on a number of factors.

Activity 4.1
What factors do you think need to be taken into consideration in planning the implementation of PBL?

Commentary 4.1
You may have identified some of the following:
Preparation of faculty staff (both academic and administration)
Preparation of students
Preparation of clinical staff
PBL team size
Selection of PBL team membership
Selection and training of PBL facilitators
How to begin the process of team building
Student roles in the PBL team
Development and selection of PBL triggers and matching programme objectives

---

Your list may include some of the areas identified above and also other aspects of preparation which are related to your own unique circumstances. The key point for you to consider is how you would tackle each area and move towards successful implementation of PBL. In this chapter we will discuss the issues related to:

- PBL team size
- Selection of PBL team membership
- The process of team building
- Student roles in PBL
- PBL and programme objectives

Selection of PBL team membership

One of the keys to successful PBL is the ability of the PBL team to function effectively in carrying out the learning activities associated with the PBL process. If the PBL team does not function as an effective unit, then students may not be developing the team skills required to be effective team players. This could be a disadvantage in the clinical setting where team work is central to the delivery of quality nursing care (Engel, 1992), and leads to improved management of client problems (Antai-Otong, 1997). The selection of PBL team membership is therefore a crucial step in the successful implementation of PBL into the curriculum.

Activity 4.2
Consider the reasons why this issue must be thought through and identify different ways in which you could select the membership of the PBL teams.

Commentary 4.2
According to Cavanagh and Coffin (1994) and Creedy and Alavi (1997) it is now the norm for cohorts of nursing students to represent a diversity of age, ability and previous nursing experience. It is therefore essential that some consideration is given to this when deciding on PBL team membership.

Engel (1992) pointed out that PBL teamwork helps develop the necessary team skills required by health care professionals. Therefore from the very beginning of a programme of study that relies on team-work, the team an

---

(Contd.)

individual finds themselves in must involve some careful consideration by faculty.

The educational journey experienced by the PBL team will have a bearing on how well students are prepared for practice. Allocation of students to PBL teams is the first stage on this journey.

You may have considered some of the following ways of allocating individuals to PBL teams:

- Branch specific groups at Foundation level
- Random allocation of all students
- An equal mix of ages, genders, educational background and branches
- Balanced team membership based on a survey students existing team skills
- Self selection

Des Marchais (1993) points out that one of the clear benefits of PBL is that it promotes team-work. Nursing is a team activity, the PBL process of education is a team activity, therefore the skills developed within a PBL team can be transferable into practice. This will only happen however if the PBL team functions effectively, team selection may go a long way to ensuring this actually happens. It is therefore important to discuss each of the options suggested in the 'commentary' in more depth.

Branch specific groups within the Common Foundation Programme (CFP)

This is probably the first decision to be made, since it is likely that at branch level the PBL team will be branch specific. The decision at CFP level will be affected by the number of branches delivered by the faculty and the very nature of the CFP component of the programme. In our experience, since the CFP is generic then it is not necessary for the teams to be branch specific provided that the triggers are directed to the issues which ensure students are exposed to material which is related to the outcomes for entry to branch (UKCC, 1999). This is essential as the majority of members of any team, simply based on the size of the adult intakes in most higher educational institutions, will be adult students. Therefore, to prevent any suggestion of bias towards adult nursing, real life triggers must be derived from all branches of nursing. This will ensure that through the use of real life triggers (not necessarily in practice), that all students are exposed to key issues related to all branches of nursing (UKCC, 1999). There are clear advantages in the common foundation programme in having mixed branch groups as this will expose all students to a wider learning experience and ensure that the generic component of the programme serves the needs of all students at the beginning level of the programme.

Once a decision has been reached regarding the make up of the teams in terms of 'branches' the next decision is the actual size of the teams.

Team size

There can be no doubt that team size is a crucial issue to be explored within any nursing faculty. Brown and Atkins (1990) examined this issue and recommended group sizes of 5 students for tutorials to 20 students for seminars. This would be supported by Fry *et al.* (1997), who suggested that small group teaching groups should be no larger than 20 students. If the teams are too large then debate and learning activities are curtailed and individuals can hide and avoid becoming part of the educational process. If the groups are too small then the work load for each student increases and more importantly the level of debate and discussion will be reduced. Belbin (2000) went further and suggested that interaction within a team leads to effective team functioning, however if the team size increases then the 'intelligent behaviour' of the team decreases.

In our experience the optimum PBL team size would appear to be 10–12 students. This may cause difficulty with facilitation dependent on intake numbers, therefore careful consideration must be given to the application of PBL within a given programme as teams bigger than this, driven only by teaching resources, may impact on the quality of the learning experience for students and lead to ineffective education and frustration for both students and facilitators.

The next question to be considered and answered is allocation of students to teams.

Random allocation

Although on the surface random allocation seems a good idea as it ensures that the team make-up is not dictated by faculty and is 'pure', it does present the possibility of teams who are unrepresentative of the real world. Simply by chance a team may not include team players who can assist with the development of team skills in others. The group may by chance be all female or all male or include a narrow range of life experiences amongst its members. In an educational context it would seem inappropriate for the make-up of what is a key educational forum for discussion, debate and the development of lifelong learning skills to be left to chance.

An equal mix of ages and sexes and branches

This is the second option for PBL team membership and is worth considering. It does require a decision on the part of faculty, with the team membership being manipulated to attain a similar balance within each team based on a 'pro-rata' breakdown of the actual cohort. This may not result in true equality in a balancing sense (e.g. each group having 5 males and 5 females each in a different age range). At a micro-level it does, however, represent the cohort of students and may be more representative of actual teams in the real world of clinical practice. A clear drawback for this option is that it does not take account of an individual's ability to function as an effective team member and therefore can and does result in dysfunctional groups (Burns, 1999). It could be argued that this is acceptable as it mirrors the real world of practice where students will encounter dysfunctional teams and need to develop strategies to overcome some of the difficulties encountered. These strategies can and are learned within the context of PBL, facilitated by an educational process which prepares students for the reality of practice.

Balanced team membership based on a survey of students' current team skills

There are many examples of the different skills required for successful groups to function together with a recognition that not everyone has these skills. (Figure 4.1 illustrates Belbin's nine team roles.) However, an effective team uses the individual strengths of all of its members in order to function effectively. Belbin (2000) suggests that careful team selection is crucial if the team is to be effective in undertaking the tasks required of it. This option takes into consideration

Plant: solves difficult problems
Resource investigator: develops contacts
Co-ordinator: promotes decision making, delegates well
Shaper: has the drive and courage to overcome obstacles
Monitor evaluator: sees all options, judges well.
Team-worker: listens, builds, averts friction, calms the water
Implementer: turns ideas into practical solutions
Completer: delivers on time
Specialist: provides knowledge and skills in rare supply

Figure 4.1   Belbin's nine team roles
(adapted from Belbin, 1993)

individual team skills and then bases PBL team membership on a mix of students who each bring their own qualities to the group. This ensures not only effective team members, but also offers weaker team players the opportunity to begin to develop team skills in the safe environment of the school prior to exposure to the real world of nursing. Belbin (1993, p. 91) suggested that in order 'to build a well balanced team that there is a reasonable supply of candidates, adequate in number and in diversity of talents and team roles'. It is therefore an avenue worth exploring if we, as educators, wish to ensure that our PBL teams are involved in 'intelligent behaviour' (Belbin, 2000, p. 44). (This is a method we are currently exploring with adult branch students at the University of Dundee. Early anecdotal evidence suggests that these teams are up and running very quickly, and with each member fufilling a key role within the team.)

Self-selection

There are some strong arguments both for and against this method of PBL team selection. The positive aspect of this approach is that it allows students to select their own team with the perceived benefit of this leading to motivation as a result of being able to select the individuals they wish to work with. On the other hand, self-selection could result in 'cliques' with an inappropriate mix of individuals who do not produce the goods. It is also worth pointing out that in the early stages of a programme, students are not aware of each others' individual traits and may have difficulty selecting which team to be a member of. There is also the possibility that one or two students are not wanted by any of the groups leading to a major problem for faculty in that a group may emerge simply because they were not popular with other students. More importantly these self-selected teams in the main will not be representative of the real world of nursing as the majority of nurses cannot select their colleges, and as this is the world of nursing for which we are preparing our students, the PBL teams must reflect this world if they are to help students to prepare to practice in it.

Bruhn (1992) noted that in comparing community staff's perception of PBL students against those taught on traditional courses, the PBL students had a more holistic view of the world and better communication and organisational skills. If this is to be the case then the first step towards this will be directly affected by the team selection. It is therefore important that this issue is fully debated and open to scrutiny. Students and academics must be fully aware of the mechanism for team selection and understand the rationale behind team selection in order to function more effectively within the team.

The process of team building

There is a general consensus that it takes time for any team to become fully functional:

Activity 4.3
Outline some reasons why this might be the case.

Commentary 4.3
You may have noted that teams take time to become fully functional for a number of reasons including the development of trust and relationship building between members, comfort in becoming a member of the team along with developing confidence, and the development of team skills.

Effective teams take time to develop and students and staff do encounter problems with the PBL approach to learning (Savin-Baden, 1997). Savin-Baden (1997, p. 531) does note however, that PBL must be seen as a 'progressive learning method'. There are, however, strategies which can be put in place to help this process along and encourage PBL teams to become effective vehicles for learning at the earliest opportunity. It is worth pointing out that part of learning for students is related directly to the process of team building. The team building skills developed as part of the PBL process are transferable into the real world of work, where effective team-working is essential in the delivery of a quality health service.

Two early strategies that are worth considering are *ice breakers and the development of PBL agreed team rules of behaviour.*

Ice breakers

It is essential that team members relax and engage with each other at the earliest opportunity, preferably before they engage on specific curriculum related PBL sessions. Therefore, the first PBL meeting should be informal and offer the opportunity to break the ice and allow students to get to know each other. Various games and strategies can be employed for this exercise (see Clegg and Birch, 1998), or why not do as we do and surf the net for ideas.

PBL team rules

There can be no doubt that for any team to function there needs to be a clear definition of rules and an agreement on how to function within the team. Faculty can take responsibility for developing these 'rules'. It is however a useful exercise in itself to allow teams to formulate their own rules as this gives the team ownership and makes the enforcement of these rules a less traumatic experience as the team has agreed to abide by them from the outset (Figure 4.2).

PBL teams who are functioning as a team are often able to recognise a clear process of 'team-building' (Burns, 1999). This is seen by Engel (1991) as a key component of successful PBL. PBL teams which function effectively are productive in developing their knowledge, and collaborate in order to work together for the benefit of the team (Engel, 1991). This was supported by Stern (1997, p. 594) who in analysing a 7-week programme for occupational therapy students, found that they felt that the PBL process had enhanced their 'responsibility to the group' and made them better 'team players'. PBL then can be an effective process, but the development of teams is an essential step which cannot be bypassed in

PBL team rules
The group must be

1. Punctual
2. Participate in the PBL approach to learning
3. Respect the opinions of others
4. Allow all team members time to speak
5. Respect confidentiality within PBL sessions
6. Endeavour to produce work within deadlines set by the team
7. Notify the team of any extenuating circumstances affecting performance
8. Ensure rotation of chair and scribe

An example of rules developed by a Common Foundation Programme PBL team

Figure 4.2   PBL team rules

the implementation of PBL. Yes, the 'real life' nursing triggers are important but time must be given for the team to become familiar with each other and decide on how they wish to organise themselves and how they expect each individual to contribute to the PBL process before the preparation for practice component is introduced.

Student roles in PBL

In order for teams to function effectively, every member must be clear as to their role within the team. People in teams need to work for and with the other team members. PBL encourages a shared approach to learning and it is important that students realise that they may be required to develop different roles within the team. PBL teams are not hierarchical in nature but do require effective organisation in order to function effectively. Team-building exercises and the development of team rules will help the members begin to appreciate the team expectations and how they, as individuals, are expected to function in the PBL team.

It is clear that during this process of team-building and role identification, that the PBL facilitator offers one avenue of support for the team but the team members must also take on some key roles within the team. Two of these roles are chair and scribe.

Chair: It is important to recognise that any team which has a function to fulfil requires organisation. If we agree that a hierarchical structure is inappropriate within PBL, we must agree that there is a need for order within the group to ensure that the team fulfils the required PBL team 'tasks'. The position of Chair then plays an important part in the structure of the team and encourages collegiate working. The Chair is therefore a position which is often rotated within the team (this ensures that individuals are offered this role as part of their own professional development). The role of the chair is to:

1. Act as a focus of control for the team meetings.
2. Ensure the team activities are related to the PBL scenario.
3. Ensure all members of the team are involved in team discussion and decision making.
4. Monitor the allocation of workload.
5. Clarify issues and help direct the discussion.

Scribe: It is unnecessary to keep minutes of a PBL team meeting. There is however a need to capture the flavour of the team discussion and record key points and decisions reached by the team. A scribe selected from the team (and often rotated), is an essential element in good team-work and management. The role of the scribe is to:

1. Keep a note of key points discussed during a PBL session.
2. Reflect this information back to the group.
3. Record the areas to be explored further and the allocation of workload to each team member.
4. To keep a group folio of information and feedback derived from each PBL session.

Students will also develop their own roles within the group and will from time to time move in and out of different roles (see Figure 4.1 Belbin's nine team roles). The student who has had a recent clinical experience in an Accident and Emergency department may become the expert and resource investigator during discussions on a PBL scenario based around emergency care. This type of 'student narrative', which is an important feature of PBL will provide illumination of how the topic under discussion fits with the 'real world' of practice. It also provides the team and the facilitator with an insight into the students' perspectives of nursing.

Students need to be clear about the PBL process and their role within the team to ensure successful PBL. The facilitator plays a key role in this, but students need to take increasing responsibility for the functioning of their team.

PBL and programme objectives

PBL is an educational process that strives to ensure that the learning which takes place is directly related to practice and that students are prepared for the reality of work. Harden *et al.* (1999) indicate that the programme objectives of any course will drive the educational options chosen to ensure the objectives are reached. If the programme objectives put great value on the recall of factual information often dictated by the assessment strategy (see Chapter 7), then the educational methods adopted will be towards the passive end of the scale and not encourage active participation in the learning process (Davis and Harden, 1999).

As nursing moves forward with the implementation of new curricula based on the UKCC (1999) recommendations contained within 'Fitness for Practice', then programme objectives must fit with PBL. If they don't, then a question must arise as to their validity as a preparation programme for tomorrow's practitioners where active lifelong learning is an essential requirement. PBL offers the opportunity for students of nursing to engage in 'active learning promoting deeper understanding and higher order thinking' (Davis and Harden, 1999, p. 8) – a worthwhile goal for all nursing curricula.

Conclusion

Barrows (1986) suggested that PBL offers the opportunity to help structure knowledge for clinical use promoting student motivation and the development of lifelong learning skills. This will happen only if some of the key issues explored within this chapter are addressed by faculty. If little thought is given to these issues then PBL will fail to deliver the goods and students will be disadvantaged during their educational journey. It is essential that curriculum planners take cognisance of this, as a thoughtful approach to PBL implementation will lay the foundations for a programme of nurse education that facilitates meaningful links between theory and practice (Burns and Glen, 2000).

References

Antai-Otong, D (1997) Team Building in a Health Care Setting, *American Journal of Nursing*, **97**(7): 48–51.

Barrows, H S (1986) A Taxonomy of Problem-based Learning, *Medical Education*, **20**: 482–6.

Belbin, R M (1993) *Team Roles at Work*, Oxford: Butterworth Heineman.

Belbin, R M (2000) *Beyond the Team*, Oxford: Butterworth Heineman.

Brown, G and Atkins, M (1990) *Effective Teaching in Higher Education*, London: Routledge.

Bruhn, J (1992) Problem-based Learning: an approach toward reforming allied health education, *Journal of Allied Health*, **212**: 161–73.

Burns, I (1999) *Problem-based Learning and Preparation for Clinical Practice: A Student Nurse's Perspective*, MSc Dissertation, RCN/University of Manchester (unpublished).

Burns, I and Glen, S (2000) An Educational Model for Preparation for Practice. In Glen, S and Wilkie, K (eds) *Problem-based Learning in Nursing: A New Model for a New Context*, London: Macmillan Press – now Palgrave Macmillan.

Cavanagh, S J and Coffin, D A (1994) Matching instructional preferences and teaching styles: A review of the literature, *Nurse Education Today*, **14**: 106–10.

Clegg, B and Birch, P (1998) *Instant Team Work*, London: Kogan Page.

Creedy, D and Alavi, C (1997) Problem-based learning in an integrated nursing curriculum. In Boud, D and Feletti, G (eds) *The Challenge of Problem-based Learning* (2nd edn), London: Kogan Page.

Davis, M H and Harden, R M (1999) *Problem-based Learning: a practical Guide*, Dundee: Centre for Medical Education, University of Dundee.

Des Marchais, J (1993) A students-centered, problem-based curriculum: 5 years' experience, *Canadian Medical Association*, **149**(9): 1567–72.

Engel, C (1991) Not just a method but a way of learning. In Boud, D and Feletti, G (eds) *The Challenge of Problem-based Learning*, London: Kogan Page.

Engel, C (1992) Problem-based Learning, *British Journal of Hospital Medicine*, **48**(6): 325–9.

Fry, H, Ketteridge, S and Marchall, S (1997) *A Handbook for Teaching and Learning in Higher Education: Enhancing Academic Practice*, London: Kogan Page.

Harden, R M, Crosby, J R and Davis, M H (1999) An Introduction to Outcome-based Education, *Medical Teacher,* **21**: 7–14.

Savin-Baden, M (1997) Problem-based Learning, part 2: Understanding learner stances, *British Journal of Occupational Therapy,* **60**(12): 531–6.

Stern, P (1997) Student perceptions of a problem-based learning course, *The American Journal of Occupational Therapy,* **51**(7): 589–96.

UKCC (1999) *Fitness for Practice: The UKCC Commission for Nursing and Midwifery Education,* London: UKCC.

5

Identifying The Issues

Introduction

This chapter aims to assist you in identifying your learning needs from the PBL scenario, organising the workload and finding the necessary information to support your recommended response to the situation. The issues that will be explored in this chapter are:

- identifying issues
- organising workload
- finding answers

This chapter is designed to be worked through like a PBL scenario. Therefore you should adopt the perspective of a nursing student in your approach to it.

Remember that PBL is not formal, teacher-led small team-work. The topic to be studied will not be taught, nor will the facilitator identify and assign tasks to be completed. It is up to you to decide what you need to learn and how you are going to achieve this. As we pointed out in Chapter 4, the environment in the PBL sessions should be confidential and non-threatening. You should feel comfortable in expressing your point of view and making suggestions. This does not imply that everything is cosy and that it's OK to produce sloppy, poorly prepared work – your team-mates will soon point this out!

Identifying the issues

Take time to examine the trigger material thoroughly. If the trigger is a video or audiotape you can ask to see or hear it again at any point in the session. Read the situation and check that your understanding of it matches that of your colleagues'. If there are differences discuss the situation and try to come to a shared understanding of what the situation is about. If you have not been given a specific situation, remember that you will need to state your position when identifying issues in the trigger, for example are you considering the trigger from the perspective of a community nurse or a nurse in the Accident and Emergency department? Are you the team leader or a junior member? Do you need to consider the roles of other people in the team?

Brainstorming: (also called thought showering)

This is a useful technique, which can help you to get started. Record all of the thoughts that occurred to you when you saw/heard the trigger no matter how ridiculous or 'off the wall' they may seem. All members of the team should contribute to give as wide a spectrum of ideas as possible. Remember that the proceedings of the PBL team are confidential. No one is going to report on how silly your suggestion subsequently proved. Ideas that appear trivial when first raised, can often lead to sound interventions when explored further. The down side of this is that no one will report on how brilliant your ideas were.

Activity 5.1
Consider the cartoon in Figure 5.1
The small boy (wee Angus) has arrived in the casualty department with his mother.
Jot down the issues that you think needs to be addressed.
Consider the situation from your current perspective or from the perspective of a D grade registered nurse (we suggest that students adopt the latter stance – it could be you one day!)
Consider your list of issues.
You have probably included some of the issues discussed below.

Knowledge:

Wound healing – how do wounds heal? What factors influence the rate at which wounds heal? How can a nurse decide if a wound is healing properly? What dressings should be used for knife wounds?

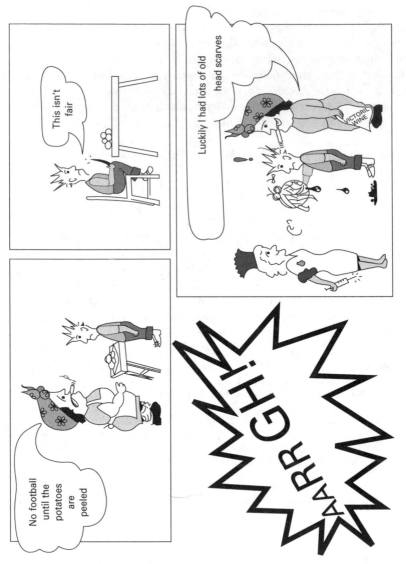

Figure 5.1   Wee Angus

Stages of child development – when does a child have the skill to peel potatoes safely using a knife?
Self-harm
What is the 'At Risk' register? How are children placed on it?
Smoking cessation – what advice should be given? What is the best method of giving advice? Is this an appropriate time to mention smoking cessation?

Skills:

Wound dressing technique
Suturing technique – (if appropriate to grade of nurse and Trust policies)
Communicating with children

Attitude:

Towards non-judgemental, reassuring, calm
Away from criticism or panic

Alternatively ....

Another way of deciding on issues to explore is to consider the feelings that the trigger provokes, then look at what you know about the situation (the facts), and decide what you need to find out (the questions or learning objectives).

Activity 5.2
Look again at 'wee Angus'.
Write down your own feelings.

Commentary 5.2
You may have been amused – the cartoon looks like something from *The Sun* or *The Mirror*.
You might have felt that it's stupid or insulting or stereotypical.
You may feel that there aren't any relevant issues at all.
You might feel dismayed – what sort of mother gives her young son a knife to peel potatoes?
Or sympathetic – imagine having to peel potatoes when you want to play football.

Activity 5.3
Now consider what feelings the characters in the cartoon might have experienced.

Commentary 5.3
What did you come up with?
Pain, guilt, fear, panic, love, concern, dismay, resentment, lack of knowledge?
Are any of these issues which the nurse would require to address in her care for Angus?

Make a note of the ones which you think are relevant. Include feelings which you thought of that are not in the list. The point of PBL is that *you* decide what you need to know, not the writers of this book or even your teachers!

Activity 5.4
Now jot down what you know about the situation.

Commentary 5.4
At first it may seem that you know very little. You don't know Angus' family name, his age or his status in the family. You are not even sure how badly he has cut himself. This is often the case when you first become involved with a patient.

On the other hand you know that somehow Angus has managed to cut himself while peeling potatoes; the wound is bleeding judging by the dripping in the picture; his mother is sufficiently concerned to have brought him to the casualty department; Angus' wound is at risk of infection – from the potatoes, possibly from the headscarves and perhaps from the hospital – there's a nurse with a large syringe to back up this feeling. His mother smokes so is risking not only her own health but also that of Angus and any other children in the family. She appears to be overweight. You also know that the wound will have to be dealt with, nursing staff will be involved at some point as it will required to be dressed.

You may be tempted to make assumptions. Perhaps Angus's mum drinks too much alcohol – she has a carrier bag from a wine shop. Perhaps she neglects Angus – otherwise he would not have cut himself. It is human nature to make judgements. As nurses we need to be aware of our responses and to take care that we are acting on fact rather than instinct. However the instinctive response may cue us into examining Angus more closely and to look for signs which may indicate neglect.

Activity 5.5

Look at the lists of feelings and facts you have produced. What do you want to know more about to deal with this situation? What do you already know?

Commentary 5.5

You may understand wound healing and have skills in dressings but need to find out more about the 'At Risk' register. You may want to find out how to communicate with children or how to begin health promotion. Only you know what you already know and can decide what you need to learn.

In a PBL team situation you will need to explain to the others why you think these are areas to be explored. This is good practice for your clinical experience. You will almost certainly be in situations where you need to justify actions such as explaining to a client why he should continue taking the prescribed medication or convincing other multi-disciplinary team members that a particular intervention is justified. Discussion with your peers will also give you an indication if your knowledge base is similar to theirs. Do they have knowledge you ought to have? Do you understand things that they don't? Can you explain things to each other?

Hopefully what you need to know to improve the given situation and what you want to learn to enable you to practice as a nurse are similar. Learning seems easier, more valuable and lasts longer when you are interested in what you are learning and are given the opportunity to apply it. In PBL you can test your learning by presenting it to other members of your PBL team and answering their questions. Later the learning can be used in clinical placements. The real test of what you learn on a nursing programme is not your mark in an examination or essay – it is your ability to apply what you have learned to clinical practice.

Activity 5.6

When you have identified your learning needs, look again at the questions to be answered. Are they clear? Do you know exactly what you are going to look for? It is worth clarifying the questions at this point, as you will save time searching if you know what you are actually looking for.

Recap:
Read/listen to/look at the trigger – several times if required.
Discuss the situation with team members.
Brainstorm the issues or consider the feelings, facts and questions associated with the trigger.
Identify what you need to learn.
Clarify the questions you need to answer.

Organising the workload

When you have decided on the questions that need to be answered you need to divide up the work. At first glance this sounds a simple exercise, but in practice it can be a time-consuming process that can create a great deal of disharmony within the team. Over time, however, you should develop people skills (which again will be useful in practice), that will assist you in working in teams and managing people (see Chapter 4).

Before you divide up the work look at any resources that have been provided for you. These vary greatly from course to course and from School of Nursing to School of Nursing. Very few nursing departments in the UK run problem-based courses that are not supported by some taught input. Most pre-registration programmes offer at least lectures and skills workshops in addition to the PBL tutorials. Several have Intranet back-up which provides, for example, lecture notes, key references, links to useful web sites and so forth. It is worth considering these resources at some point in the work allocation process. If the whole class is timetabled for a lecture on the physiology of wound healing, should this be a topic for exploration or is it expected that every member of the team will contribute to discussion on wound healing in the feedback session? Are there specific aspects of wound healing related to the PBL scenario which merit particular attention? Will each member access all the Internet material on smoking cessation or can one member summarise it and feedback to the others? Do you all need to visit the local social work department to ask about the 'At Risk' register or are there other approaches? You will probably find that at least some of the issues you identified from the trigger will be addressed in other parts of the course. Be prepared to integrate this learning into your response to the PBL trigger.

Trust

Members of the team need to rely on each other to do the work and produce the resources required. Where there is a lack of trust, some team members will try to cover all aspects of the scenario and others will do very little work. You will gain more from PBL if you divide the learning fairly equally among the team members. Inevitably there will be differences between scenarios resulting in one or two members having a heavier workload for that scenario. The team, guided by the chair, should endeavour to ensure that it is not always the same people who take on most work. This may not be easy to assess when you are new to PBL. Sometimes it can be difficult to predict how much effort will be required to research a particular topic. It will be easier to allocate the work fairly if you make sure that each of you is clear about the questions you want answered. Time spent in the team focusing on the questions will save time when you come to search for relevant material. As a team member you have the responsibility for ensuring that you are pulling your weight and that other members are contributing. (Reasons for non-participation and how to deal with it are covered in Chapter 7.) You will gain more from PBL if you select a different aspect in each topic. For example, if you have a particular interest in anatomy and physiology, try not to select this element from every trigger. Perhaps you could select a sociological or environmental issue instead. Similarly, if you have been able to negotiate your choice of topic in every PBL session, try to sit back and encourage one of the quieter members of the team to speak out and get the topic they are interested in, instead of deferring to the more vocal members of the team. If you are one of the quieter members, plan in advance how to get in your say. Your facilitator will encourage the team to evaluate its performance on a regular basis (see Chapter 8). This is an opportunity for you to say how you feel – for example that you always get left with the topic no one else wants or that everyone else always expects you to cover the life sciences. Expect to contribute to the discussion on how this can be overcome in future sessions.

There is no need to manipulate the material to give each member one issue. Some triggers will create lots of small issues, others trigger two or three large issues. The team may decide to work in pairs or threes if the topic identified seems too big for one person and cannot be split up logically. Try to ensure that you do not always work with the same person(s). It is comforting to work with people you know well, but this will not always happen in practice. You need to develop the skills to get on with different types of people. You may already have worked in clinical areas where certain staff like to work together. How comfortable was this for the other staff?

When you have defined and negotiated your learning issue, identify times when you will work on it. Lack of time will lead to superficial searching and surface learning, therefore you will very quickly forget what you have learned. As mentioned earlier, the main purpose of problem-based learning is not to help you pass the assignments (although it should do that too!), but to provide you with the knowledge you need to be a qualified nurse or midwife. To be a competent practitioner you not only need to know what to do but also why you are doing it.

Finding the answers

Just as there may be supporting lectures and workshops, you may also be provided with reference lists, URLs and names of experts who are willing to be contacted. As you become more experienced, it is likely that the resources you are given will be reduced and you will have to start seeking the material for yourself.

Activity 5.7
Go back to the list of issues you identified in the 'wee Angus' trigger. Pick two or three that interest you.
You have no reference list and no supporting teaching – where would you find the information you want? Write down the sources you have identified.

Commentary 5.7
Probably your list looks something like this:
Library – books and journals
         – University library, local library
The Internet
Videos
Leaflets/pamphlets
Self help teams/help lines etc
Social Work Department
Health professionals – nurses, GPs, health visitors
You now need to decide which of these resources is best suited to answering your questions.

Book and journals – searching the literature

In PBL you will need to find the best evidence to inform your thinking. The first step in this process is to search the literature. 'Literature' generally refers to material that is published, with no judgement made as to its quality. Making a judgement on the value of an article or book, 'critiquing', is an essential skill for nurses and midwives (ENB, 1998). It takes time to develop the ability to read critically. This skill is beyond the scope of this book.

Most pre-registration courses and many post-registration/graduate programmes include critical reading as a component of the course, often as part of a research module. Some universities also run critical reading courses for students in addition to the sessions within the programme (there may be a charge). Investment of time and effort in acquiring critiquing skills will bring rewards in the form of increased understanding and enjoyment in reading research reports and improved judgement of which innovations could usefully be applied to your practice (not to mention better grades in assignments!).

You may find that your facilitator encourages you to find material from articles, preferably where the writer of the article is the person who has carried out the research (these are termed primary sources). Utilising the original research allows you to explore the author's own meanings rather than obtaining the results second-hand (secondary sources), when they may have been subjected to someone else's perspective prior to publication. Textbooks are useful, but the length of time between writing and publishing the text may mean that material is not always up-to-date. However the explosion of nursing literature following the move of nurse education into higher education in the 1990s has also extended the publication times of journal articles. Textbooks usually supply extensive reference lists and thus can be a source for material by using the 'author' category in databases to seek recent publications by the authors referenced.

There are several other types of journal in addition to the primary journals (*Journal of Advanced Nursing, Nurse Education Today*), and journals such as *Nursing Times* and *Nursing Standard* that provide nursing news coverage in addition to professional articles. These include review journals, professional journals and controlled circulation journals. Review journals such as the *Nursing*

Clinics of North America provide summaries or updates on specific topics written by experts. The summaries usually include extensive reference lists. Similar to review journals are abstract journals that provide abstracts not only from published research but also reports, theses and work in progress. Professional journals tend to target practitioners rather than researchers. Often the focus of the journal is a particular area of nursing such as Care of the Elderly or Critical Care. They aim to keep practitioners up to date with the latest best evidence practice. Some professional journals have controlled circulation, in that they are available only to individuals who work in a particular speciality who often are members of a particular organisation and receive the journal as part of their subscription, for example the Association for Continence Advice. Libraries may carry some of these. You may find that others are available in clinical areas related to the speciality.

Additionally, information can be obtained from reports produced by agencies such as the Nursing and Midwifery Council (NMC) and the Chief Scientists' Office. Such reports include information that may be omitted from journal articles such as the detail of research tools used. Circulation of reports may be restricted to people with a particular interest in the topic and hence it can be difficult for others to obtain a copy. The growth of the Internet has improved access to reports, as many organisations will place a copy of commissioned reports on their web sites. Theses undertaken as part of a higher degree area are also valuable sources of information, demonstrating originality of thought and providing full detail of research methodology and results. Material from theses can be hard to access, as you need to know that the material exists before you can access it. Theses may only be available for consultation in the library of the university where the research was supervised. It may be that some of the material from a thesis has been presented at a conference, therefore published papers from conferences can be a rich source of information.

Remember that some of the topics you identify may be found in journals other than nursing. In the 'wee Angus' trigger in this chapter, for example, you may find that you can obtain required information from social work journals.

To find out what has been published on the topic that you have identified you will need to search through this vast amount of material. Although it is still possible to search material by hand using nursing/midwifery indexes, this tends to be a long and laborious process. Computerised databases such as CIHNAL and Medline have made the search for writing on a topic quicker and easier. Contact your own school or departmental library for help. For novice searchers using databases is sometimes too easy, resulting in thousands of references. As stressed earlier in this chapter, the tighter and more focused your question, the more clearly you will be able to define your search terms and thus will be less likely to end up with large numbers of titles.

Sometimes the reverse happens and there are apparently no articles on your subject. If this happens to you, try to think of words with similar meanings. If you get stuck your library should have a book called a 'thesaurus' that will give you alternative words. Many word-processing packages also have this facility. It may also help to keep notes of the original brainstorming session for the trigger. As you become more familiar with the databases you will find the process gets easier. If you find yourself totally unable to proceed ask a PBL team member, your facilitator or a member of the library staff for help. PBL is about helping you to learn not only the knowledge you will require to become a nurse but also the skills that will help you keep your practice up-to-date when you are working as a qualified nurse. Literature searching is one such skill. When you have a manageable number of sources, decide which ones are key, for example articles that have been recently published or present information in an understandable format. Unless you are convinced that an article is really valuable, choose journals that are held locally or that can be obtained quickly from another library. The time between the introductory session and the feedback session is usually too short to obtain copies from other libraries. Copies can also be costly. Remember that you may be able to access journals electronically via your library web pages. Specialist units may hold journals related to their speciality. While they are unlikely to allow you to borrow them, many areas are sympathetic to a polite request to peruse the journals on site. Likewise other schools, departments or faculties in the university may allow you access, but not lending rights, to their department libraries. Related material may be available in medical or law schools, other health-related professions such as occupational therapy, physiotherapy, dietetics or social work, education departments. Local community libraries will have information on local issues, for example census figures for the local area, maps, local history, self-help teams (see below). They may also hold newspaper archives.

Using the Internet

The World Wide Web also provides access to a vast selection of material. The process of selecting material from the Internet has been likened to 'drinking from a waterfall with a teaspoon'. The amount of information available is vast. Like the databases a single search term may result in thousands of 'hits' or none at all. Redefining of search terms may be necessary. Unlike published material, which will have been subjected to scrutiny ranging from that of a single editor to review by panel of experts prior to being printed, anyone can post almost anything on the Web. Sites owned and run by organisations such as the Department of Health, the Royal College of Nursing or the NMC provide reliable information. Be aware that sites which may appear reputable can contain information that is little more than personal opinion, for example university sites may contain personal Web pages that reflect the views of individual lecturers based on unsound or even no research. On the other hand it is often useful to have insight into individual opinions on conditions, treatments and so forth as this will assist you in caring for patients with these conditions. Personal accounts of dealing with illness or disability can also be helpful. Be critical of the material you choose. Apply the knowledge you develop from your research sessions in selecting which pages to download. Course tutors and Intranet sites often provide guidance on finding relevant sites.

Steps in the search

Make sure your question is well focused

⇓

Identify key terms from your question

⇓

Conduct search

⇓

Redefine terms if necessary

⇓

Select relevant sources and print out

⇓

Retrieve articles from stock or find Web page

⇓

Read to decide most relevant

⇓

Copy relevant articles

⇓

Critically read and synthesise for feedback

⇓

Create reference list for the team

While the greatest emphasis is placed on evidence obtained from published material, information about the PBL topic being explored can be obtained from other sources.

Non-literary sources

Videos/CD-ROM

Visual material is often a useful resource. Demonstration of a particular procedure, presentation of case studies and interviews with experts or patients can often be obtained on video.

Other organisations

Organisations such as the Health Education Boards hold a range of material and will send out photocopies on request. Again there will be a moderate charge and it may take some time for the information to reach you. It is helpful if you can focus your request as much as possible to assist in locating the material. Self-help and charity organisations such as Chest, Heart and Stroke, the Mastectomy Association and Age Concern often have information in the form of leaflets or copies of relevant articles, many of which

are free. The purpose of these organisations is to improve understanding of the disorder for suffers and their carers. Many organisations will be willing to provide you with their material as part of
the dissemination of information, but you may be asked to contribute to postage and packing. The information is often available
on a web site, so it is worth checking first. It is preferable that only
one person from the PBL team approaches the organisation and
that representatives from several teams make contact jointly.
Patient and carer support groups are often willing to talk to students. Statutory and local government agencies such as social work
departments, local housing authorities and rights offices will also
have information that may relate to some of the PBL triggers with
which you may be presented. Information may be available in
leaflet form and readily obtainable. If you need more detailed
advice, try to arrange a suitable time in advance. Staff in such agencies have considerable claims on their time. Although they may be
willing to assist you, remember that this is not their main function.
Several agencies such as the Benefits Agency and Local Police
Departments often provide information that is held by the school
library.

Experts

Lectures and tutorials will give you an insight into the interests of
the teaching staff in your School of Nursing. Teaching staff may be
willing to give you more information or point you towards suitable
resources. Information can also be obtained from mentors in the
clinical area. Once again if you are not actually attached to a men-
tor while investigating a PBL topic, we suggest that you arrange a
suitable time in advance. Teaching staff may be able to advise
which clinical staff, for example specialist nurses or medical staff,
are willing to talk to students. Contact numbers may be given as
part of the resources that support the PBL scenario. These are
busy people and may not have time to talk to you. Again it may be
helpful for one or two students to approach clinical staff and then
share the information with the others. Teaching and clinical staff
can provide information on best practice and how it is applied in
a particular area. One of their main strengths lies in providing
insights into the lived world of nursing, answering questions that
tend not to be addressed in textbooks or articles for example

'which grade(s) of nurse would look after "wee Angus" and when would a doctor be involved?' 'Why are some nurses able to suture and some aren't?'

Finally, recognise that PBL team members as individuals have a great deal of information that may be relevant. It is likely that at least one of your colleagues has had a placement in casualty or has had to take a young relative to the Accident and Emergency department. Sharing experiences and discussing feelings and reactions to situations can provide increased awareness and insight.

Summary Activity
List the issues you identified from the storyboard of wee Angus
Reflect on the process that led you to produce this list
Note the resources you decided to use to learn more – do you know how to access them? If not find out.

Reference

English National Board for Nursing, Midwifery and Health Visiting (1998) *Developments in the use of an evidence and/or enquiry-based approach in Nursing, Midwifery and Health Visiting Programmes of Education,* London: ENB.

6

Encouraging Critical Thinking Through PBL

Introduction

This chapter will examine how PBL offers students the opportunity to develop the skills required for critical thinking. We agree with Paul and Heaslip (1995, p. 40), who suggest it is essential that nurses develop 'the ability to think critically about the knowledge required for care and the knowledge she brings to the nursing care situation'. In our opinion PBL offers students of nursing the opportunity to develop these critical thinking skills.

Activity 6.1
How does PBL encourage the development of critical thinking skills?

Commentary 6.1
You may have identified some of the following:

PBL is a process that encourages education through facilitation which helps students develop critical thinking skills by providing the opportunity to explore and develop 'knowledge' which is relevant to practice.
Organising and presenting material requires the student to engage in a higher level of thinking than traditional teaching methods.
The need for students to integrate other aspects of the curriculum to inform their decision making, feedback and discussion.
PBL provides greater opportunity to question and explore students' thinking.
The need to engage in reflective practice.
PBL encourages students to link their learning to the knowledge and skills required for effective nursing practice.

However this process does not just happen, it needs to be managed effectively to ensure students are given the opportunity to explore their own knowledge base and develop aspects of critical thinking. We will discuss how this can best be achieved by exploring issues related to:

● Facilitation
● Questioning
● Reflection
● Integrating fixed resource sessions
● Organising and presenting material

Facilitation

The role of the facilitator in PBL is central to the success of a PBL curriculum (Happell, 1998; Schwartz *et al.*, 1997 and Stern, 1997). According to Happell (1998, p. 364) the PBL facilitator's role is 'not to provide information in response to students questions but to assist them to discover what they need to know'. This is supported by Stern (1997), who points out that the facilitator's role is about giving the students guidance in order to allow them to take responsibility for their own learning.

Activity 6.2
Think about your own teaching practice or the teaching practice of lecturers you have come in contact with and identify some of the qualities of an expert PBL facilitator.

Commentary 6.2
In considering the issues surrounding expert facilitation you may have identified some of the following attributes of an effective PBL facilitator. PBL facilitators:

● enable students to take responsibility for their learning
● encourage team interaction
● challenge assumptions
● act as a role model
● act as a resource person
● are willing to empower students
● have an enthusiasm for learning
● scaffold student learning (see Chapter 8)
● encourage respect and mutual trust within the PBL team

Little (1997) suggests that the path from lecturer to facilitator of learning, within the context of PBL, is often an 'uneasy one' (p. 121). As Little (1997) goes on to point out, it is often the case that lecturers value themselves as subject experts and, according to Drinan (1997), are in-post because of that expertise and not because they have expert facilitation skills. Oliffe (2000) goes further by suggesting that without preparation most academic staff do not possess expert facilitation skills. What is also clear is that subject expertise does not in itself prepare academic staff for PBL facilitation. It is clear however that the success of PBL is in itself dependent upon academic staff having facilitation skills and understanding how to adapt to the PBL process (Oliffe, 2000).

If the path from expert lecturer to expert facilitator is not completed then tutor problems identified by Holmes and Kaufman (1994) and expanded on by Rono (1997) may become an issue for faculty. Rono (1997) identified these tutor problems when carrying out a small study into the challenges and limitations of PBL within a medical school in Kenya. Rono (1997) identified tutor problems such as 'inexperience', 'tutor domination' and 'negative attitudes'. Facilitators must be able to engage with students as individuals to ensure the smooth running of the PBL session, students in our experience consistently report that facilitator interest in them is very important and motivates them to engage in the PBL process. Skilful facilitation is a key component of successful PBL (Creedy and Alavi, 1997). If PBL facilitators do not adopt a truly facilitative style then tutor problems will impact on student learning and the development of lifelong learning skills which promote critical thinking. We would therefore agree with Albanese and Mitchell (1993), who suggest that PBL may be more successful when delivered by an enthusiastic small group of lecturers. It is good practice to expose as many lecturers as possible to the PBL process. It may however be more beneficial to target committed enthusiasts to actually carry out the PBL facilitation, thus ensuring the students are truly facilitated through the PBL process.

It is evident therefore that students must be encouraged to analyse their current nursing knowledge and how their learning will enhance their next nursing experience (Paul and Heaslip, 1995). In a PBL context this can happen only through expert facilitation which encourages students to challenge themselves and their peers in developing 'new knowledge' which directly impacts on practice.

Questioning

A key component of effective PBL facilitation worth exploring separately is questioning. Effective questioning during the PBL process is essential if students are to be encouraged to move beyond conversations about nursing and develop analytical skills which will encourage them to question and learn through questioning.

Activity 6.3
Explore why questioning has a key role to play in a PBL process which encourages the development of critical thinking skills.

Commentary 6.3
It is likely that you have identified that questioning is often the first and most important aspect of engaging in critical discussion within the context of PBL. Asking questions allows individuals to clarify the salient issue related to the PBL scenario and begin to explore their current knowledge and where gaps in that knowledge may exist. It is therefore a crucial component of any PBL session. You may have also discussed the fact that there are different types and levels of questioning. Questioning may also arise from the PBL facilitator or from within the team, the purpose being to help each member of the team to think clearly about the issues generated during the PBL session. This will lead to team members engaging in 'intellectual effort' allowing them to develop knowledge which is directly related to practice situations (Paul and Heaslip, 1995).

It is therefore worth exploring the concept of effective questioning as without it, PBL will be ineffectual and may dissolve into a negative learning experience for all team members. House *et al.* (1990) explored this concept and clearly outlined the reasons why questioning is an essential element in effective teaching. It encourages students and facilitators to engage in a 'teaching moment' which can challenge and stimulate learning, direct the thinking process, encourage discussion and help the students to evaluate their learning.

It is clear that the more complex the questions asked the more demand will be placed on the PBL team members. Bowling (1979) cited by House *et al.* (1990) outlined three levels of questions:

- knowledge questions
- application questions
- problem solving questions

Students and facilitators should be encouraged to explore the types and levels of questions that could be used within a PBL context. As aspects of questioning can be explored before a PBL session begins, it is possible to ensure that effective questioning technique is utilised to maximise student learning (House *et al.*, 1990). Although students should be encouraged to develop their questioning skills, expert facilitation requires the facilitator to have considered the true purpose of questioning and explored the components of effective questioning.

A key component of effective questioning is the development of listening skills. PBL team members must be prepared to engage in effective communication skills, one of which is the ability to listen. Listening strategies are crucial to the development of critical thinking skills and team participation in the learning process. Inappropriate listening skills can lead to problems within the team, leading to aspects of 'disjunction' and ineffective team behaviours (see Chapter 7). It is essential that team members listen to each other and provide appropriate verbal and non-verbal cues that encourage individuals to engage in responding to questions and participate in effective communication. Non-verbal communication plays a key part in effective facilitation during the PBL process. Students become adept at reading facilitators' body language and following the signals. Therefore along with a strong line in questioning the facilitator must ensure that nods, smiles and noises such as 'u-huh' and 'mm-hum' encourage students to proceed with a line of thought. Frowns or a lack of response provoke a change of topic or silence. Non-verbal communication such as 'over to you' gestures and the rolling of hands to 'keep going' can be used to keep students in discussion if the facilitator feels that further questions or spoken engagement might disturb the process.

Team members must also be made aware that making mistakes is acceptable. Teaching and learning is a two-way process which can be enhanced during PBL by effective questioning and listening. Strategies adopted by the facilitator and team members must prevent student withdrawal and positively encourage full participation by all team members in what is a very active approach to learning. This approach will facilitate a more effective approach to deeper learning than more traditional teaching methods. Students will engage in an 'inquisitive style of learning rather than rote learning' ensuring that the knowledge created is directly applicable to the practice situation (Magnussen *et al.*, 2000, p. 360). This is supported by Barrows and Tamblyn (1980) who recognised that the most important skills required in clinical practice are problem solving skills and not memory skills. This inquiry approach to learning where the facilitator facilitates learning and does not lecture will strengthen the students ability to engage in critical thinking (Magnussen *et al.*, 2000).

Reflection

Paul and Heaslip (1995, p. 41) suggest that student nurses begin to think critically when they realise that they must continually answer the question 'what do I really know about this nursing care situation and how do I know it'. This process of reflecting on one's current knowledge base is crucial for active PBL, leading to an increasing awareness about a person's current knowledge needs.

Activity 6.4
Consider the benefits that active reflection can bring to increasing critical thinking through the use of PBL.

Commentary 6.4
You may have identified that reflection is a means which will help team members to develop personal and professional knowledge. PBL allows students the freedom to engage in discussion and debate about real nursing situations, while reflection encourages students to engage in a process which can lead to meaningful learning. This process then encourages the student to examine their knowledge and skills in the light of what knowledge and skills are required for practice.

In the real world of nursing you may have already noted that you do not always have time to stop and reflect on a given care situation. PBL, in dealing with real nursing issues, gives the student the time to reflect-on-practice and learn to think critically about practice.

Taylor (2000, p. 11) in discussing reflection, suggested that 'the ability to think in a systematic and rational way separates humans from other species and gives people reflective consciousness'. This critical thinking process is therefore a key component of reflection and, we would suggest, a skill which must be developed if the student wishes to engage fully in the PBL process. The level of thought processes required will however be dictated by the level of challenge presented to the student at any given time. It is therefore essential that the level of challenge within the PBL is directly related to the level expected of the student within their programme of study.

In order to engage in reflective practice it is essential to understand the basic premise surrounding reflection, which is that through reflection an individual can develop their 'personal, practical and intuitive knowledge' (Smith *et al.*, 2000, p. 2). Students must also be able to utilise an effective model for engaging in reflective practice. Although there are a number of reflective models available such as Gibbs (1988) *Reflective Cycle* and Johns (1995) *Model for Structured Reflection (10th version)*, we introduce our students to the Marks-Maran and Rose (1997, p. 14) reflective cycle (Figure 6.1) which helps give structure to the process of reflection.

The process of reflection in conjunction with PBL will therefore engage the student in a model of learning that will encourage them to develop their critical thinking skills by:

- analysing the situation presented in the scenario
- establishing current knowledge and skill levels
- identifying gap areas in both knowledge and skills
- discussing and debating as a team how to resolve the issues presented
- engaging in a process which encourages both personal and professional development

This process of PBL and reflection will allow students of nursing to identify 'the difference between the knowledge and understanding one brings to a new situation and the knowledge and

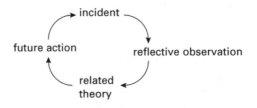

Figure 6.1   Marks-Maran and Rose's reflective cycle

understanding one takes away from a new situation' (Marks-Maran and Rose, 1997, p. 120). The aim is to create new knowledge and skills and encourage the use of reflective and critical analysis skills. PBL and reflection together will encourage the student to engage in more complex thinking which will lead to a critical approach to learning (Taylor, 2000).

Integrating fixed resource sessions

In most nursing courses and programmes which incorporate PBL there are fixed resource elements which support the PBL within any given term. In the early terms of our pre-registration programme within the University of Dundee, PBL is supported from fixed resource session from areas such as:

- nursing communication
- nursing assessment and care planning
- nursing core skills
- biological sciences
- social sciences

This type of approach is supported by Albanese and Mitchell (1993), who do not advocate a total PBL approach to curriculum design. We would agree with Schwartz *et al.* (1997) who note that there is still an important role for other teaching methods, including didactic teaching, in a PBL curriculum. It is however essential that a PBL curriculum which is supported by fixed resources must function in such a way that is cohesive and the fixed resources support and are linked to the PBL component of the curriculum.

Students must be able to recognise the clear links between the fixed resources and PBL, and be able to relate the information back to the challenges posed by the PBL sessions. This is a key component of effective PBL – students must be receptive to the links and may at an early point in their programme need positive help in developing these links. If we can encourage students to develop these skills then we will allow them to become 'active creators rather than passive receptors of knowledge' (Glen, 1995). When these links are made by students then the knowledge and skills which form part of the fixed resource sessions will become real for

the student. It is essential in a curriculum which is based on PBL
to ensure the learning is integrated. Therefore there must be
a clear relationship between the fixed resources and the PBL
scenarios (Ryan and Lyttle, 1991).

Activity 6.5
How would you ensure that students are able to integrate the fixed
resource session into the PBL process?

Commentary 6.5
You may have identified that it is essential that curriculum planners have
clearly defined the purpose and function of fixed resource sessions
within the programme and that students are aware of their purpose. They
should provide the student with additional material which will assist with
their learning (Wilkie, 2000). Students should then be encouraged to
synthesise the information covered within these sessions and select the
information needed to engage in the feedback aspect of the PBL process.

Fixed resources can take a variety of forms:

- lectures (compulsory/optional/student request)
- tutorial
- clinical skills session
- open/distance learning
- computer assisted learning
- journals/books/videos
- personal interviews
- clinical experiences

In planning the curriculum it is essential that faculty fully consider their approach to fixed resources within a PBL curriculum.
The number and content of these types of sessions varies across different programmes of study. The guiding principle must however
be one of supporting PBL and therefore engaging the student in
the PBL process. Lectures, for example, need not as in the past
cover 'all the material' required in a given area of study, but focus
on the key concepts and relate these to the PBL the students are
engaged in at that point in time (Armstrong, 1997). As Wilkie
(2000, p. 18) points out we must avoid the pitfalls of a 'belts and
braces' approach to PBL which dilutes its principles. Students
must be encouraged to be active in their learning, not exposed to

a passive process which devalues self-directed study, with fixed resource sessions providing the answers the lecturer thinks the students need. This would undermine the principles of PBL and will not encourage critical thinking and deeper learning (Wilkie, 2000). We support the ideas expressed by De Bono (1967) that it is better to be skilled in thinking than to be stuffed with facts. Fixed resources should not detract from encouraging active student learning but support the PBL learning process. Students will benefit greatly from thinking through the issues involved in nursing for themselves and sharing these thoughts with the PBL team. This will encourage understanding and reduce their reliance on the 'expert' lecturer to provide the solutions (Fisher, 1988).

Organising and presenting material

The final session in a structured PBL timetable is the feedback session where students are required to engage in feedback, discussion and debate. This final step in the PBL process must allow the students, through expert facilitation, to organise and present material which enhances students learning and the development of 'critical thinking' skills.

Activity 6.6
Outline why the prospect of organising and presenting feedback is often challenging for students.

Commentary 6.6
You may have identified that nursing attracts a wide variety of entrants, which means that we have to 'address a wider range of abilities than any other discipline' (Creedy and Alavi, 1997, p. 219). Some students may feel threatened in an educational environment which requires them to become fully participative from the very beginning. As a result of different backgrounds, students may not have been exposed to an educational system which requires them to be challenged to organise and present material to their peers.

It is important that prospective students are made fully aware of the requirements of PBL and are facilitated to develop the skills required to organise and present material to the PBL team. It is also important that when selecting students for nursing programmes which are designed with a PBL component, that selected students have 'the potential to benefit from and succeed in such an environment' (Long and Grandis, 2000, p. 64). We would also suggest that if students cannot function in this type of environment then they will be unable to function in the real world of nursing where we require practitioners who are adaptable and responsive to change – 'in short are capable of life long learning' (Candy, 2000). We must ensure that we do not set students up to fail, but encourage and facilitate their development to ensure they can develop critical thinking and life long learning skills.

Students will require help in developing the skills required to organise their study activities related to PBL. In a traditional approach to learning the organisation of the sequence of learning is often left up to the curriculum planners and/or the individual lecturer. The actual content of each session is therefore organised for the student with the decision between 'what is important and what is unimportant' made for them (Davis and Harden, 1999). The organisation of student learning is managed for the student and taken out of their control. In PBL, students are encouraged to do this for themselves in terms of exploring the problem scenario, identifying the issues and how to tackle the learning activity. The development of the problem scenarios is therefore a crucial step in helping the students to organise their thinking and indicating the amount of student activity which may be required. We agree with Margetson (1997), who suggests that PBL forms a focus for student learning activities which will expand their understanding of, in this case, nursing practice. The PBL problem scenarios must lead the student into an area of meaningful learning related to practice and should be driven by and focused on practice. This will help the students to not only develop organisational skills in learning but also in the delivery of appropriate evidence based nursing care.

Once students have organised their learning activities and the information they need to gather, the next crucial aspect of effective PBL is the presentation of material to the team. This presentation must focus on the problem scenario and possibly on wider issues related to taking this developing knowledge and skills into clinical practice. In the same way that it is desirable to use different types of trigger material in designing problem scenarios, it is also advisable to devise learning activities which require the student to engage in different ways of presenting material to the team. The presentation of material must maintain group interest and generate discussion and debate which ensures that all team members participate in the learning process.

Activity 6.7
Brainstorm the different mediums that could be used to present material to the team.

Commentary 6.7
You may have identified some of the following:

- verbal reports/supported by written material
- flipchart material
- acetate presentations
- power-point presentations
- slides
- videos
- role play
- nursing documentation
- debate

Students should be encouraged to explore different modes of presentation, to prevent PBL sessions deteriorating into no more than mini-lectures delivered by each team member, which do not challenge the students to learn. The student activities outlined within the problem scenario may also help focus their thoughts on the type of presentation expected by the team. When teams are at a beginning level the problem scenarios may give clear indication of the expected type of feedback often related to the type of information sharing which occurs in practice situations. This may include care plans or handover reports rather than just a 'verbal essay' on care delivery. PBL is based on reality, therefore feedback should prepare students for the reality of communication in nursing practice. Although students may take time to develop their presentation skills, this development period should be facilitated in a similar way to other skill development within a nursing programme. This process of development must be accepted by both facilitators and students as through time 'the regular expectation placed on students to present to their peers using a range of approaches reinforces group cohesion and increases confidence' (Long and Grandis, 2000, p. 63).

Conclusion

Garratt *et al.* (2000, p. 153) suggest that 'in developing the skills of thinking, it is clear that one must have something to think about'. We suggest that PBL gives the student 'something to think about' and encourages the development of critical thinking skills through a process of facilitation in dealing with issues related to the real world of nursing practice. PBL exposes the student to a learning process which encourages the development of key 'thinking skills' which according to Garrett *et al.* (2000, p. 154) are:

- analysing and evaluating arguments
- making judgements
- retrieving information
- experimenting

PBL will help develop nurses who are not only lifelong learners but professionals who are critical thinkers able to broaden their base of nursing knowledge and help shape the future of health care delivery.

References

Albanese, M and Mitchell, S (1993) Problem-based learning: A review of the literature on its outcomes and implementation issues, *Academic Medicine,* **68**(1): 52–81.

Armstrong, Elizabeth, G (1997) A Hybrid Model of Problem-based Learning. In Boud, D and Feletti, G (eds) *The Challenge of Problem-based Learning* (2nd edn), London: Kogan Page.

Barrows, H S and Tamblyn, R (1980) *Problem-based learning: An approach to medical education,* New York: Springer.

Bowling, B (1979) *Questioning: The mechanics and dynamics.* Lexington: University of Kentucky, Teaching improvement project system. In House, B M, Chassie, M B and Bowling Spohn, B (1990) Questioning: An essential ingredient in effective teaching, *The Journal of Continuing Education in Nursing,* **21**(5): 63–8.

Candy, P C (2000) Reaffirming a Proud Tradition: Universities and Lifelong Learning, *Active Learning in Higher Education,* **1**(2): 101–25.

Creedy, D and Alavi, C (1997) Problem-based learning in an integrated nursing curriculum. In Boud, D and Feletti, G (eds) *The Challenge of Problem-based Learning* (2nd edn), London: Kogan Page.

Davis, M H and Harden, R M (1999) *Problem-based Learning: a practical guide,* Dundee: Centre for Medical Education, University of Dundee.

De Bono, E (1967) *The Five Day Course in Thinking*, Oxford: Oxford University Press.

Drinan, J (1997) The Limits of Problem-based learning. In Boud, D and Feletti, G (eds) *The Challenge of Problem-based Learning* (2nd edn), London: Kogan Page.

Fisher, A (1988) *The Logic of Real Arguments*, Cambridge: Cambridge University Press.

Garratt, J, Overton, T, Tomlinson, J and Clow, D (2000) Critical thinking Exercises for Chemists: Are They Subject Specific?, *Active Learning in Higher Education*, 1(2): 152–67.

Gibbs, G (1988) *Learning by Doing: A guide to teaching and learning methods*, Oxford: Further education Unit, Oxford Polytechnic.

Glen, S (1995) Towards a New Model of Nursing Education, *Nurse Education Today*, 15: 90–5.

Happell, B (1998) Problem-based learning: providing hope for psychiatric nursing?, *Nurse Education Today*, 18: 362–7.

Holmes, D B and Kaufman, D M (1994) Tutoring in problem-based learning; a teacher development process, *Medical Education*, 28: 275–83.

House, B M, Chassie, M B and Bowling Spohn, B (1990) Questioning: An essential ingredient in effective teaching, *The Journal of Continuing Education in Nursing*, 21(5): 63–8.

Johns, C (1995) Framing Learning Through Reflection: Eithin Carper's Fundamental Ways of Knowing in Nursing, *Journal of Advanced Nursing*, 24(4): 226–34.

Little, S (1997) Preparing Tertiary Teachers for Problem-based Learning. In Boud, D and Feletti, G (eds) *The Challenge of Problem-based Learning* (2nd edn), London: Kogan Page.

Long, G and Grandis, S (2000) Introducing Enquiry-based Learning into Preregistration Nursing Programmes. In Glen, S and Wilkie, K (eds) *Problem-Based learning: A New Model for a New Context?*, London: Macmillan.

Magnussen, L, Ishida, D and Itano, J (2000) The impact of the use of inquiry-based learning as a teaching methodology on the development of critical thinking, *Journal of Nursing Education*, 39(8): 360–4.

Margetson (1997) Why is Problem-based Learning a Challenge. In Boud, D and Feletti, G (eds) *The Challenge of Problem-based Learning* (2nd edn), London: Kogan Page.

Marks-Maran, D J and Rose, P (1997) *Reconstructing Nursing: Beyond Art and Science*, London: Bailliere-Tindall.

Oliffe, J (2000) Facilitation in PBL-espoused theory versus theroy in use: reflections of a first time user, *The Australian Electronic Journal of Nursing Education*, 5(2).

Paul, R W and Heaslip, P (1995) Critical Thinking and Intuitive Nursing Practice, *Journal of Advanced Nursing*, 22: 40–7.

Rono, F (1997) A students' review of the challenges and limitations of problem-based learning, *Education for Health*, 10(2): 199–204.

Ryan, G and Lyttle, P (1991) Innovation in A Nursing Curriculum: A process of Change. In Boud, D and Feletti, G (eds) *The Challenge of Problem-based Learning*, London: Kogan Page.

Schwartz, R W, Burgett, J E, Blue, A V, Donnelly, M B and Sloan, D A (1997) Problem-based learning and performance-based testing: effective alternatives for undergraduate surgical education ansd assessment of students performance, *Medical Teacher*, **19**(1): 19–23.

Smith, L, Bruce, B, Clarke, G, Denovan, D, Gall, Tulloch, L and Venters, A (2000) *Partnerships in Learning Module Workbook*, Dundee: School of Nursing and Midwifery, University of Dundee.

Stern, P (1997) Student perceptions of a problem-based learning course, *The American Journal of Occupational Therapy*, **51**(7): 589–96.

Taylor, Beverly, J (2000) *Reflective Practice: A Guide for Nurse and Midwives*, Open University Press: Buckingham.

Wilkie, K (2000) The Nature of problem-based learning. In Glen, S and Wilkie, K (eds) *Problem-Based learning: A New Model for a New Context?*, London: Macmillan – now Palgrave Macmillan.

7

Managing Team Dysfunction and Disjunction

Introduction

The success of PBL depends on the ability of the team to function as a vehicle for shared learning. As with any active team approach to learning, if the students do not play as a team then team dysfunction is the likely outcome. This will result in ineffective learning and ultimately poor preparation for practice. It is therefore essential that one considers the possibility that PBL will challenge students to utilise 'team skills' (see Chapter 4) in order to undertake effective learning.

This chapter will explore a number of issues, which could, if not handled properly lead to dysfunctional teams. The issues to be explored are:

- disjunction
- frame factors
- institutional assessment strategies
- non-participation of team members/poor attendance at PBL team meetings.

Disjunction

Disjunction within an educational context has been defined as 'a sense of fragmentation of part of, or all of the self, characterised by frustration and confusion, and a loss of sense of self' (Savin-Baden, 2000, p. 87). This can lead to a feeling of loss and frustration for the student in the context of a PBL approach to learning.

This is particularly true if students are seeking clarity in the learning process and a 'teacher/student' relationship where the 'teacher' is the expert who will always provide the correct answer or a solution to the students learning needs. Taylor and Burgess (1997, p.108) go further and suggest that disjunction for some students can lead to 'trepidation and outright terror' as they approach an unfamiliar educational experience such as PBL. This, they argue, is particularly the case for students with a non-traditional entry route into higher education. As the entry gate to nursing has 'widened' it has to take account of the fact that many of its undergraduates will enter via non-traditional routes and need to learn how to become active participants in the learning process. They will have to adapt quickly to 'modern' approaches to active learning within the higher education sector.

Activity 7.1
Explore some of the reasons why students may experience disjunction when exposed to the PBL process.

Commentary 7.1
You may have identified some of the following reasons:

- self-direction in the learning process may be new to the student and present them with a challenge in adopting unfamiliar patterns of learning behaviour
- role conflict may occur if the student is unfamiliar with a process that gives ownership of knowledge creation to the student rather than a process that sees the student as a receptacle for the teacher's knowledge
- students may become frustrated with a learning process that does not provide them with the correct answer on demand
- students often come unprepared for the unique challenges presented by PBL
- students who are not confident in themselves often feel threatened in a setting that requires them to actively engage in a team based approach to the learning process.

It is therefore essential that both academic staff and students face these issues. If unresolved they will lead to frustration and anger in both camps and a failure to use an effective PBL approach to learning. Savin-Baden (2000) would argue that disjunction is inevitable when adopting PBL and we all face it at some point during this learning process. The key however is to be positive and recognise that disjunction is 'not unhelpful and damaging' (Savin-Baden, 2000, p. 87), but instead can be used in a positive light to move students forward in the development of themselves as learners. This enables the student to become more self-aware of their individual learning needs and how to adapt their learning style to ensure they have the lifelong learning skills required to practice as a nurse in an ever-changing health care environment. This active approach to learning is supported by Candy (2000) who considers that there is clear evidence available which suggests that active learning approaches, including PBL, provide students with the skills necessary to engage in continual learning throughout their professional career.

There are barriers to learning in any learning situation. Within PBL it is important to recognise these barriers, and in particular disjunction, and adopt strategies to overcome them, enabling the students to grow as learners. It is therefore essential that both the PBL facilitator and the team members create a learning environment which supports the transition of the team through this process, seeing disjunction as a issue to be dealt with as a team for the ultimate benefit of the team. It is important that in doing so, the PBL facilitator and team value each other's contribution, recognise the different qualities each individual brings to the team and invest time and energy in effective team-building (see Chapter 4). Disjunction can and will occur, but if viewed as a positive learning experience it can be used to enhance learning and team functioning. In our experience if disjunction is met head-on by all team members it brings the team closer together as a functional learning unit, where all members feel they have something to contribute to a facilitated peer-assisted approach to learning. A learning approach that in reality reflects how learning takes place 'especially in professional and work related contexts' (Candy, 2000, p. 114).

Frame factors

Jacobsen (1997) in a study of medical students on a problem-based undergraduate programme, found that students often brought what he termed 'frame factors' to PBL meetings. He defined a frame factor as an issue not related to the PBL scenario being studied, but of importance to the team or some team members. Frame factors in Jacobsen's study usually related to events, which had occurred during the students' clinical experience. Facilitators tried to steer students away from these issues, back to the PBL scenario, usually with little success. The most commonly occurring frame factors raised by nursing students were assessments (this issue will be examined separately), and issues related to practice placement allocations.

Frame factors can permeate the PBL session and prevent the students from engaging with the PBL material.

Activity 7.2
Outline reasons why students would bring these 'frame factors' into a PBL team meeting.

Commentary 7.2
Once the PBL team has become established it provides a regular point of contact for students. The PBL sessions tend to lend themselves to the development of an effective peer support mechanism, allowing team members to share experiences and discuss and debate their clinical and academic encounters in a safe educational environment.

Facilitators sometimes tend to view frame factors as irrelevant as they are perceived as having nothing to do with what students ought to learn. However as frame factors have the potential to severely disrupt a PBL meeting, facilitators need to develop methods of dealing with them as students find it difficult to put unresolved issues out of their minds. The opportunity provided by frame factors therefore must be capitalised upon and not ignored. If we wish to engage our students in active learning, then it is possible to use the introduction of frame factors in a positive way to enhance the PBL experience for the students involved.

One method of dealing with frame factors is to set a time limit for discussion of topics not associated with PBL. Another is to encourage students to raise their own issues during PBL. There is, however a risk that PBL meetings will become counselling sessions, although some students may find this beneficial and appreciate this level of support. It may be more appropriate with some frame factors, which are clearly related to an individual's life experience of nursing, to take these issues outside the PBL team and deal with them on an individual basis. This will ensure that the student or students are directed to the relevant person or department for appropriate support and guidance.

In our experience, with the exception of clinical experience, frame factors become less of an issue as students progress through their programme of study. The fact that frame factors related to clinical practice experience continue to be raised throughout the students' programme has led to some facilitators setting aside time during the PBL meeting to allow students to reflect on their clinical experience, in any module which follows a practice placement experience. Although, for some, this may not seem part of the remit of PBL, it is akin to 'student-generated' PBL, which ensures that student issues related to the real world of practice are taken cognisance of and given an airing. This then not only develops the PBL teams' cognitive and reflective abilities, it ensures that PBL team members feel ownership of the team processes. According to Davis and Harden (1999) one of the aims of PBL is to allow students to take an increasing level of responsibility for their own learning. Facilitating the team to explore specific frame factors as part of the PBL process helps students to take ownership of aspects of the PBL process and deal with issues that are real to them. This, when the issues have been discussed, then allows the team to move on and concentrate fully on the PBL task in hand.

Institutional assessment strategies

The purpose of this section is not to present an exhaustive list of assessment strategies that are compatible with a PBL approach to curriculum design, or to discuss and debate the merits of different assessment strategies for PBL. For in-depth discussion and debate we would refer you to Nendaz and Tekian (1999), Marks-Maran and Thomas (2000) or Rideout (2001). However we have included some examples of assessments we have employed to reduce the conflict between assessment and the active approach to learning advocated by PBL (Figures 7.1, 7.2 and 7.3).

This section will examine the disjunction that can arise within a student when there appears to a be conflict between what is being asked in the context of PBL (a strategy that encourages students to

The aim of this assignment is to enable the student through participation in the assessment of a chosen client to further develop assessment skills and to reflect upon the assessment process.

You should select, from your current placement, a client who will be the subject of your assignment. This assignment will enable you, through close interaction with your chosen client (and where possible a significant other), to gather bio-psychosocial data. This data will assist you to identify a range of nursing problems or health needs.

Guidelines

1. Introduce your client giving a brief inroduction to his/her background and the reason for his/her admission to the ward/nursing home.
2. Select and briefly describe an appropriate nursing assessment framework.
3. Using your chosen framework carry out and subsequently describe in your essay the information gained from the assessment of your client's nursing problems/health needs.
4. Select and describe an aspect from the assessment that requires more specific assessment.
5. Describe briefly how you would consider carrying out a more specific assessment of this aspect of the client's nursing problem/ health needs.
6. Where appropriate, research based material should be utilised to support any assertions made.
7. The final part of the essay should draw together your findings.

Total wordage: 2000.

N.B.
The selection of your client should be undertaken in consultation with your preceptor/mentor. It is important that you ensure confidentiality by using a pseudonym and not the client's real name. You should state that a pseudonym is being used. At no point in the essay should you reveal any information that would identify anyone involved in the client's care or the identity of his/her significant others.

Copyright School of Nursing and Midwifery, University of Dundee.

Figure 7.1   Year One: nursing assessment

develop self-directed learning skills in order to create solutions to 'problems'), and what is being asked by the assessment strategy adopted by the institution. As indicated earlier when discussing frame factors, one of the most commonly occurring frame factors for nursing students is assessment. This is not surprising as assessment and evaluation of learning, even in traditional courses, is a

This assessment will take the form of a structured essay, the Nursing Issue chosen will be derived from the one of PBL sessions explored in module 10.

Guidelines

- In consultation with your PBL facilitator choose a nursing issue related to one of the PBL sessions in Module 10.
- You are required to carry out an in-depth study of the nursing issue chosen and present a structured essay.
- The essay should have a clear Title, Introduction, Main Body of Text, Conclusion including Recommendations (if appropriate) and a Reference List.

Total wordage: 2500.

Copyright School of Nursing and Midwifery, University of Dundee.

Figure 7.2   Year Two: problem-based learning essay

source of conflict. This is not helped by the fact that at times there is little agreement between PBL enthusiasts on the most effective method of student assessment within a PBL curriculum (Rideout, 2001 and Swanson *et al.*, 1997).

Activity 7.3
Identify aspects of institutional assessment that in a PBL context may lead to disjunction between learning activities encouraged by PBL and the assessment strategy adopted by the institution.

Commentary 7.3
We would expect you to agree with the fact that PBL encourages team-based activity learning facilitated by the discussion of real-life events and the integration of subject matter (Marks-Maran and Thomas, 2000). This promotes critical analysis leading to application of knowledge in the real world of nursing (Rideout, 2001). This then leads to the issue of whether or not the assessment strategy adopted by the institution encourages and promotes this type of learning. If the only assessment strategy used is focused on subject-based learning with little or no integration across subjects or into clinical practice, then this will inevitably lead to disjunction and dysfunction both at team and individual level. It may lose the profession the type of graduate who has the ability to take on board the concept of lifelong learning and make a significant difference in clinical practice. It could actively discourage the development of transferable and lifelong learning skills.

'Critical incidents are a way of examining a particular situation in your practice and identifying what you have learned from it. "Critical" here refers to your critical examination of the situation.' (Girot, 1997, p. 48)

For this assessment you are required to:

Choose a situation from recent practice; using a model for reflection reflect on your experience of the situation; identify and discuss the issue(s) it raises; draw conclusions regarding your learning from the process of reflection.

This assignment is designed to encourage you to analyse and 'reflect-on' practice. It is therefore essential that you protect the identity of any individual or areas involved.

Guidelines

- Select an incident.
- Identify the model for reflection and type of reflection you are undertaking.
- Reflect on your role in the event and the effect it had on you.
- Focusing on one issue which is of particular interest to you, analyse and discuss the literature on the subject.
- Suggest ways of applying research evidence to alternative management of the situation in the future or utilise the current research to analyse how this situation was managed effectively.

This critical incident analysis will demonstrate that you:

- are able to use the process of reflection and discuss its value.
- can appraise current practice in light of personal experience, and a comprehensive review of the literature.
- have identified your own individual learning needs.
- have conducted a coherent argument/discussion.

Total wordage: 3000.

Copyright School of Nursing and Midwifery, University of Dundee.

Figure 7.3   Year Three: critical incident analysis

How then does a PBL approach to learning and assessment match with a profession that clearly demands certain competence of its new practitioners prior to registration? This, in our view, does not compromise the PBL philosophy but can inform the development of PBL scenarios and the assessment strategy to ensure they are directed at the development of skills, attitudes and knowledge required for practice. Any professional programme of study demands of its graduates a knowledge and skill component that prepares them for practice. PBL offers this and more. The key is to ensure that when assessing both theory and practice that PBL is not ignored and students are aware that not only the acquisition of knowledge but also their developing PBL skills will be assessed. This is supported by Rideout (2001) who recognised the fact that in a profession where knowledge is important then it must be assessed. As long as the students are prepared and informed about the context of assessment within the curriculum, then disjunction related to assessment should be reduced. The key is that knowledge is learned in the context in which it will be applied and from time to time it is assessed in that context. This, in our experience, reduces disjunction and helps students engage in an active approach to learning and assessment. If this does not happen then the self-directed learning skills developed by the student 'will have as much substance, in the eyes of the students (and others) as the fabled emperor's clothes' (Norman, 1997, p. 266).

Therefore it is acceptable to include Multiple Choice Questions (MCQs) in the assessment strategy, but one must also incorporate PBL focused assessment. A balanced, and according to Norman (1997, p. 266), an 'intelligent' approach to assessment is the key. We often demand more of students (see Chapter 1) following a PBL curriculum. This reflects the reality of clinical practice where more and more is being demanded of the nurse. A PBL curriculum with a well thought out assessment strategy has the ability to prepare the student for the real world of nursing practice.

In developing our assessment strategy for our pre-registration nursing programme we adopted a mixed approach to assessment that also includes the use of simulated patients within the context of an Objective Clinical Skills Examination (OCSE). This ensures that not only are students prepared for practice but the assessments themselves are fit for purpose and match a PBL approach to learning and assessment. Figures 7.1, 7.2 and 7.3 give examples of assessments used at different parts of our programme to not only encourage the development of learning skills, but to help the student to relate the assessment strategy to the PBL process, encouraging them to deal with the reality of nursing. Ensuring that the assessments require more than rote learning and factual recall from the student, this approach encourages deeper learning that is a key component of PBL (see Chapter 2), encouraging the student to recognise this and the relevance of PBL in a learning context (Davis and Harden, 1999).

It must however be pointed out that this does not always result in a more comfortable experience for the student. When one moves out of the 'comfort' zone of a teaching and learning strategy which is focused purely on knowledge-based assessment, and into one which is more than teaching for exams then the challenge for the student is increased. There is more responsibility put on the students to select the context of their assessment and ultimate learning. This in itself challenges both the student and the academic in the PBL context. However, this then becomes an enabling process where the discussion is focused on the challenge presented by the assessment and not around the issue of whether or not the assessment takes into account the PBL process and the assessment of learning skills developed as a result of the PBL process. The time is then spent on preparation for the completion of assessments not the substance of an assessment, which is in conflict with a PBL approach to learning. The discussion and ultimate completion of the assessment is then a journey, which enhances the knowledge and skills of the student and is not an automatic process of 'testing' knowledge and then moving on. Norman (1997, p. 265) points out that assessment 'steers student learning'. It is our role to ensure that it is being steered in the right direction and we keep the students on board preparing them for a 'lifelong learning' career in nursing.

Non-participation of team members/poor attendance at PBL team meetings

Nursing and nurse education has undergone rapid change since the introduction of Project 2000 in the early 1990s, and the increasing demand for graduates/diplomates who are 'autonomous, capable of rational thought and able to make their own assumptions and decisions' (Biley and Smith, 1998, p. 1021). There has been an increasing move away from the traditional approach to nurse education which was based on a training model which relied heavily on experience gained in the 'hospital setting' (Burns and Glen, 2000) backed up by a teacher centered approach to education (Biley and Smith, 1998). This approach to teaching and learning has been credited with encouraging a passive approach to learning that does not equip the student with the educational skills required to continue to adapt and maintain professional competence in the real world of practice (Nendaz and Tekian, 1999).

Activity 7.4

In this new world where PBL is a focus for nurse education, consider why this student-centred approach to learning may lead to students opting out of the education process.

Commentary 7.4

As already discussed in earlier chapters, PBL challenges the student to be active in the learning process and for some this can be an uncomfortable process which challenges their belief systems related to the purpose and function of education. It is therefore essential when selecting undergraduates for a PBL based curriculum that there is no hidden agenda and students are fully informed about the programme, what they are signing up for and how this will equip them with the knowledge, skills and attitudes to function in an ever-changing health care environment. We must ensure we do not set students up to fail.

One of the first questions therefore that must be asked of students who are not participating in the PBL process, is why? If it is related to their discomfort with the PBL process and/or nursing, or their inability to work as a team player then one would have to examine, with them, their commitment to nursing and the development of the lifelong learning skills required of a nurse in the 21st Century. In many ways this is a relatively straightforward process and can be dealt with through discussion between the PBL facilitator/personal tutor and the student.

However, in our experience the more difficult issues are related to team functioning (see Chapter 4). It is the role of the facilitator to help the team function as a vehicle for effective learning, ensuring that the interactions are positive and helping the group achieve its goals (Wilkerson, 1995). If this is not happening then the PBL facilitator must take a lead in resolving the conflicts within the group that may be leading to non-participation and non-attendance. Conflict and disjunction within a PBL team can often arise out of unproductive relationships between individual students (student problems) or as a result of overall dissatisfaction with the performance of the PBL facilitator (tutor problems) (see Chapter 4). If this happens then it is not unsurprising that it is often followed by poor attendance and non-participation by individual team members.

It is recognised that an individual's ability to function as a team player is often attributable to a confusion over the purpose of the team and where they fit into the team (Antai-Otong, 1997). If this becomes apparent within the team then it is time to revisit through open discussion within the team the purpose of PBL and the role of the student and facilitator in this process (see Chapter 4). It is also worth reminding the team of their agreed team rules (see Chapter 4). This is often time well spent as it allows the team to examine its successes and failures, identifying what led to these successes and how can it build on this to move the team forward and come to a greater understanding of the assets the team has rather than focus on the negative. Any time invested in team building is time well spent (see Chapter 4). The problem should never be ignored or any non-attendee written off without some exploration of the cause of the disjunction as it may lead to more disruptive and dysfunctional behaviour by all team members. This may lead to displays of such behaviour as 'aggression, competition, hostility, aloofness, shaming and blaming' (Antai-Otong, 1997, p. 50). This can only result in the development of a fully dysfunctional team where there is no trust and the learning process grinds to a halt. The key is to follow the advice of Savin-Baden (2000) and change this disjunction from disabling to enabling through a process of expert facilitation.

Conclusion

Managing team dysfunction and disjunction is a reality of PBL and poses a real challenge for both students and facilitators. In this chapter we have explored a number of issues that need to be taken into account when preparing a PBL curriculum to ensure that both students and facilitators are fully prepared for engagement in the PBL process. These issues should never be ignored but resolved for the benefit of the team, individual students and the ultimate goal of preparing nurses for the reality of clinical practice.

References

Antai-Otong, D (1997) Team Building in a Health Care Setting, *American Journal of Nursing*, **97**(7): 48–51.

Biley, F C and Smith, K L (1998) 'The buck stops here': accepting responsibility for learning and actions after graduation from a problem-based learning nursing education curriculum, *Journal of Advanced Nursing*, **27**: 1021–9.

Burns, I and Glen, S (2000) A New Model for a New Context? In Glen, S and Wilkie K (eds) *Problem-based Learning in Nursing: A new model for a new context?* London: Macmillan Press – now Palgrave Macmillan.

Candy, P C (2000) Reaffirming a proud tradition: universities and lifelong learning, *Active Learning in Higher Education*, **1**(2): 101–25.

Davis, M H and Harden, R M (1999) *Problem-based Learning: a practical guide*, Dundee: Centre for Medical Education University Of Dundee.

Girot, A E (1997) Reflective Skills IN Maslin-Prothero, S (ed) *Bailliere's Study Skills for Nurses*, London: Bailliere Tindall.

Jacobsen, D Y (1997) *Tutorial Processes in a Problem-based Learning Context.* Unpublished Thesis Department of Education, Trondheins: Norwegian University of Science and Technology.

Marks-Maran, D and Thomas, B G (2000) Assessment and Evaluation in Problem-based learning IN Glen, S and Wilkie K (eds) *Problem-based Learning in Nursing: A new model for a new context?* London: Macmillan Press – now Palgrave Macmillan.

Nendaz, M R and Tekian, A (1999) Assessment in Problem-based Learning Medical Schools: A Literature Review, *Teaching and Learning in Medicine*, **11**(4): 232–43.

Norman, G R (1997) Assessment in problem-based learning, In Boud, D and Feletti G (eds) *The Challenge of Problem-based Learning* (2nd edn), London: Kogan Page.

Rideout, E (2001) Evaluating Student Learning In Rideout, E (ed) *Transforming Nurse Education Through Problem-Based Learning*, Sudbury: Jones and Bartlett.

Savin-Baden, S (2000) *Problem-based learning in Higher Education: Untold Stories*, Buckingham: The Society for Research into Higher Education and Open University Press.

Swanson, D B, Case, S M and van der Vleuten, C P M (1997) Strategies for student assessment. In Boud, D and Feletti, G (eds) *The Challenge of Problem-based learning* (2nd edn), London: Kogan Page.

Taylor, I and Burgess, H (1997) Responding to 'non traditional' students: an enquiry and action approach. In Boud, D and Feletti, G (eds) *The Challenge of Problem-based Learning* (2nd edn), London: Kogan Page.

UKCC (1999) *Fitness for Practice*, Report of the UKCC Commission for Nursing and Midwifery Education, Chairman Sir Leonard Peach, UKCC London.

Wilkerson, L (1995) Identification of skills for the problem-based tutor: student and faculty perspectives, *Instructional Science*, **22**: 303–15.

8

Evaluation of PBL

Introduction

In contrast to the previous chapter that discussed the assessment of student learning with respect to PBL, this chapter addresses the issue of evaluation in problem-based curricula. Whereas assessment centres on students and their learning, evaluation covers wider issues including those of teacher performance, course content and organisation. Evaluation can be used for a variety of purposes. Evaluation has three main purposes – to validate, thus justifying the activity and providing a rationale for its continuance, to improve by building on acceptable practice and to condemn through the highlighting of poor practice and inadequate processes. All of these purposes apply to problem-based curricula. This chapter focuses on the evaluation of student and facilitator processes within the PBL seminar and the overall evaluation of PBL as a learning and teaching strategy within the curriculum. It is not only the PBL processes that require to be evaluated. The resources available to support learning and the suitability of accommodation for PBL sessions and study should be evaluated. Evaluation of organisational issues such as the amount of time allocated to PBL and the appropriateness of the scenarios to the programme being studied is also required. The chapter does not address issues associated with the evaluation of materials related to PBL, which was discussed in Chapter 3.

It is the view of the authors that evaluation of the PBL process should be formative and qualitative. This reflects our stance with respect to PBL as a strategy that aims to foster deep learning and critical thinking skills rather than the acquisition of knowledge for assignments. However, as there are situations where it may be desirable for performance in the PBL seminar to be evaluated formally and quantitatively, this approach will also be discussed.

Evaluation of PBL performance

A note of caution must be given about evaluation of PBL performance. At first reading, evaluating seminar performance may appear to have more in common with assessment rather than evaluation. The philosophy of PBL emphasises learning for learning's sake, rather than learning in order to pass assessments, therefore formal, summative rating of behaviour in PBL seminars can be counter-productive. There is a risk that students will become more concerned with how they are performing in terms of how often they intervene or the leadership attributes they display, to the detriment of learning about the issues raised by the scenario. The PBL seminar thus becomes an exercise in facilitator-pleasing, rather than an opportunity to engage in dialogue and to develop critical thinking skills. Allocation of marks or grades for performance in seminars may be employed as a method of ensuring that all students participate during the seminar. However, the interference this creates with the PBL process may outweigh any benefits from increased participation. If there is competition for good grades among students in a PBL team, the processes necessary for team functioning, such as sharing of information, constructive criticism and supporting of members, can be lost in the desire to outperform other team members. If the overall performance of the team is graded, dissatisfaction with PBL and team dysfunction may ensue (see Chapter 7), particularly if students who are more ambitious think that some of the others in the team are jeopardising their grades.

While this argument suggests that the PBL process should not be assessed, part of the role of the facilitator is to provide evaluation about student performance in PBL seminars and the quality of the material produced by students in support of learning. Schwartz *et al.* (2001) stated that prompt, honest feedback is an integral requirement of using PBL. Issues need to be dealt with as they arise. Students should be given regular feedback on content and process in a safe environment. Time for evaluative feedback must be allowed for when scheduling PBL sessions.

Evaluation of seminar performance can be undertaken in several ways. The method selected for the evaluation will depend on the way in which the institution has elected to implement PBL (see Chapter 1). Although this section includes examples of both quantitative and qualitative methods of evaluation, course organisers are advised to consider the appropriateness of each of these to their own programmes.

Considerations in evaluating performance in PBL seminars

Evaluation of performance can be daunting for even the most experienced teacher. Facilitation of PBL is a new role for many teachers, which requires time to become comfortable. Students may find PBL daunting to begin with and may be uncertain about the level and type of performance expected of them. One of the first decisions to be made in evaluating PBL is what to evaluate. As indicated above, the learning that takes place as a result of PBL, is the product or output from the members of the PBL team, and is most commonly judged through the institution's formal assessment system. Evaluation in PBL is concerned with the process within the sessions and the contribution of the students (and facilitator) to the process.

Activity 8.1
What do you think requires to be evaluated within a PBL seminar?

Commentary 8.1
Elements frequently regarded as essential to the progress of a PBL seminar include: participation by all team members, mutual respect, willingness to challenge ideas and concepts, equity of effort and motivation to learn. Some of these elements relate to the students, however some are equally applicable to the facilitator.

Chapter 7 discusses ways of dealing with dysfunction and disjunction and team processes that have gone awry. However, processes that seem satisfactory also need to be evaluated. Questions that need to be answered in this category focus on team members' performance and the process of the seminars. Elements necessary to the PBL process include the contribution of individual students to the overall work of the team, behaviours which are helpful or unhelpful, reflection on performance, assistance to develop desirable behaviours and the application of learning to the practice setting. In the PBL situation, the evaluation of performance should to be specifically geared to each individual team and its members rather than being applied across an entire class. Each team will respond in different ways. The characteristics and attributes of the team need to be taken into account. Each PBL team will be influenced by the culture, educational background and previous experience of the individual students in the team. The academic level of the students in the programme requires consideration when evaluating the level of discussion by the team. The degree of cohesion within the team and their expertise with PBL will have an impact on the workings of the team. Facilitators need to be aware of and take account of these individual differences and responses in order to engage with the team and provide the support necessary for that team. Facilitation needs to be flexible and adapted to the needs of each individual team. Therefore, evaluation, as part of facilitation, also requires to be flexible and individualised to the team and its members.

Activity 8.2
You have identified the elements to be evaluated.
What are the other considerations in planning evaluation?

Commentary 8.2
Other considerations are linked to the organisation of the evaluation, these include

Individual student performance or team performance?
How often will evaluation take place?
Who will undertake the evaluation – facilitator, peers, students themselves or outsider?
Will the evaluation cover both student and facilitator performance?
What format will the evaluation take?

Individual performance or team performance?

Decisions about evaluating performance on an individual or a team basis are linked to the underpinning philosophy of the curriculum, how the evaluation is undertaken and who will carry out the evaluation. The format selected for evaluation should match this decision. If evaluation is undertaken through administration of a questionnaire to the whole cohort, individual evaluation cannot be provided. It is, however, possible for individual evaluations to be combined to provide an overall evaluation of a team or class.

How often?

Evaluating performance in PBL, like other evaluation, requires advance planning. Programme requirements may set specific times for summative evaluation, particularly with respect to the organisational aspects of PBL. Formative evaluation, designed to be cumulative and to assist students in building on previously identified strengths, occurs as the team progresses. Facilitators may decide that the team has reached a point where evaluation would be beneficial. Sufficient time is required for evaluation. Evaluation is rarely done well when the team members want to go to the next class or go home. Similarly, evaluation may not be appropriate after a seminar which students have found difficult or upsetting. Time for reflection may be advantageous.

Who should undertake the evaluation?

Evaluation of PBL, like most other evaluative processes, can be carried out by the individual participants on themselves (self-evaluation), by each other (peer evaluation), by/on the facilitator (by the students or another facilitator) or by someone outside the situation (external evaluation). None of these formats is exclusive. It may be of value to combine the formats or to utilise different formats at different points in the programme. Honest and realistic self-evaluation is an aim of PBL. In nursing and midwifery programmes, it is usually linked to the development of reflective practice. Using reflection-on-practice (Schön, 1987), students are encouraged to remember incidents from practice, to identify research linked to the incidents and to consider the implications for future practice. PBL provides a safe environment in which to practise this activity. Chapter 6 referred to the use of reflection within student feedback. Reflection can be used to encourage students to consider not only their own performance but also that of other members of the team and the facilitator. Students are encouraged to think back on their recent performance in the PBL seminar, evaluate their performance and consider which aspects, if any, need to be improved. Students can be given questions for consideration to help focus their thinking (see Figure 8.1). If a quantitative evaluation is required, the questions can be used in conjunction with a rating scale.

Similar questions to those in figure 8.1 can be used to assist teams to peer evaluate. Developing this reflective process and the associated beginnings of critical thinking, requires courage, skill, understanding and respect for self and others (Wolff, 1998). Difficulties encountered in promoting reflection tend to lie at two extremes. At one extreme, students may be overly critical, at the other they may not be sufficiently critical. In the first example, students can underestimate themselves and fail to recognise that the work they have produced is valuable and worthwhile. Students may be hypercritical of peers. Alternatively students may

---

Consider the questions below to help you assess your performance in PBL.

1. Did I help others to explain their ideas?
2. Did I explain my own ideas well?
3. Did I listen attentively to other team members?
4. Did I try to understand what others were saying?
5. Was I willing to challenge other people's ideas?
6. Did I give in too quickly when opposed?
7. Did I initiate discussion?
8. Was I overly aggressive?
9. Was I too sensitive to other people's feelings?
10. How relevant were my contributions?
11. Was I more often disruptive than constructive?
12. Was I too quiet?
13. Did I appear to believe people?
14. Was I too eager to express my view?
15. Was I willing to support other people's ideas?

after Newcastle Medical School, 1985

Figure 8.1 Evaluation of performance in PBL

experience the 'tyranny of niceness' (Robinson, 1995). Here the students state that everyone in the PBL team has performed well and has brought back suitable material. No challenges are made to team members and no questions are asked. These 'nice' students can be more difficult to facilitate than teams that evidence some dysfunction as the reluctance to reflect critically on self or peer behaviour inhibits the identification of how performance could be improved.

Modelling of reflection on practice by the facilitator can be useful in helping students to develop ways of giving and receiving constructive evaluation. Students report that this aspect becomes increasingly important as they approach qualification and the realisation that they will have to evaluate students and other staff in their role as qualified nurses. Evaluating peers is an activity with which students often feel uncomfortable, particularly if there are negative aspects in the evaluation. One of the limitations of PBL as preparation for team working in practice is that, other than the facilitator, all the members of the PBL team are equals, a situation that rarely occurs in clinical settings. Dealing with the content of feedback (see Chapter 6) may be easier than evaluating a colleague's contribution to the workings of the team as negative aspects can be attributed to the difficulty of the topic, the lack of published material or problems with accessing resources, rather than to individual behaviour. The issue becomes even more sensitive when evaluation is qualitative rather than quantitative as scores or grades are seen to be more objective than comments.

Evaluation by the facilitator may be regarded as the least uncomfortable format, possibly because it will be familiar to most students. Students expect to be evaluated by teachers. Most of the students will have had experience of teacher evaluation at some point before starting the programme. Evaluation can, of course, be undertaken by an external person. This is easier where quantitative evaluation is employed. Questionnaires can be administered by members of support staff, independently from teaching staff. Obtaining qualitative evaluation is more difficult. The addition of another person into the PBL team will inevitably alter the team dynamics. The observed behaviour of the team and the facilitator may differ from the norm. However, an evaluation that does not actively involve the students will not help students to develop the ability to evaluate their own performance.

Will the evaluation cover facilitator performance as well as student performance?

If PBL is promoted as a student-centred strategy, should students evaluate the facilitator? It can be argued that the facilitation role in PBL is to guide and support students in their learning. If this is the case, it seems reasonable that the people best placed to evaluate the performance of the facilitator are those receiving the facilitation. Dolmans *et al.* (1994) and de Grave *et al.* (1998) reported on facilitator evaluation within an undergraduate medical programme in The Netherlands. Using a Likert scale, Students rated facilitators on a series of characteristics including the helpfulness in guiding the learning process, the facilitator's knowledge base of the topic being discussed and the commitment of the facilitator to the team. The score given to facilitators was taken into consideration when deciding tenure and promotion for academic staff. Facilitators who consistently failed to achieve a pre-determined score, were offered remedial help. Wolff (1998) suggested that students require different approaches to facilitation at different stages in their programmes, an observation that has been supported by research with our students (Wilkie, 2002). Students who were new to PBL appreciated an approach that was directive, created comfort within the team and displayed interest in the students as individuals. As students developed PBL skills, they began to prefer a less interventionist approach that allowed them to explore freely the issues they identified from the scenario. The time taken for student teams to arrive at this point varied considerably. Facilitators who adopt a less directive approach with novice students may be poorly rated by them but well rated by more experienced students. A 'motherly' approach that may be too smothering for third year students, is often appreciated by first year students unsure of the demands of the course. Inexperienced students may also find it difficult to comment freely on a member of staff who is in close contact with them. It could be argued that the best person to carry out evaluation of facilitator performance is another facilitator, through a peer review.

Wider issues for evaluation

Although the conduct of seminars and the associated performance of students and facilitators within seminars are of prime importance, evaluation of other aspects of problem-based curricula is also required.

Activity 8.3
List other aspects of the curriculum that you would want to evaluate.

Commentary 8.3
Probably you listed organisational elements and resources such as timetabling and accommodation issues, library access and the relevance of the PBL scenarios. Some of these issues can be perceived as being of lesser importance to teachers whose main focus is student learning. However, frequent timetable changes or lack of supporting material can be frustrating for students who are often trying to balance demands such as home, family and part-time work with the requirements of the programme. Issues of timing and resourcing are important. Lack of time, shortage of materials and inadequate access to databases are frustrating and will inevitably have an impact on the quality of learning achieved through PBL.

Evaluation of facilitators has been discussed with seminar evaluation. However, as students cite facilitator interest in them and in the topic as an important element in PBL, it can also be raised within the wider context of course evaluation.

Questions that might be asked in relation to wider issues include:

Timing

Was the amount of time allocated to PBL seminars sufficient? Too much? Not enough?
Was the distribution of time between seminars sufficient for the work to be completed?
Was enough time allocated for study?
Was the PBL trigger introduced at an appropriate time in the timetable?

Relevance/Links

Did the learning stimulated by the PBL trigger match learning from other sources such as clinical skills laboratories, lectures, open learning/e-learning materials?
Was the problem-based learning relevant to clinical practice?

Resources

Were there sufficient library-based resources?
Were 'expert staff' available and willing to speak to you?
Could you easily access the Internet/Intranet?
Was there suitable accommodation available for seminars and study?

Facilitators

Did your facilitator attend all sessions?
Did your facilitator appear interested in your learning?
Was your facilitator sufficiently well-informed to assist you?

Questions of this type can readily be incorporated into a questionnaire where response is sought as either yes/no or as Likert scale format 'always/sometimes/never'. This category of items will highlight problems in resourcing and timetabling. The addition of a 'free response' section has the advantage of offering students the chance to identify problems that may not have occurred to the programme planners. Although these questions are typically asked of students, it is worthwhile raising them with facilitators at facilitators meetings. Facilitators are often aware of difficulties with timing and resourcing and can offer advice and examples of how such problems may be resolved.

Format of the evaluation

The format used to evaluate seminar performance should reflect the purpose for which evaluation is being undertaken. If the main reason for evaluation is to support student learning and to provide prompt, on-going comment on performance, a qualitative, informal style of evaluation, based on facilitator observation and notes will be more appropriate than evaluation based on a rating system. In contrast, information from evaluative questionnaires may be required to justify continuing with a particular programme. If more detail is required, for example, *why* particular aspects were rated as unsatisfactory or otherwise, other methods of evaluation may be more appropriate.

For factual information, questionnaires may be the most suitable form of evaluation. Questionnaires are widely used as they provide a quick and relatively user-friendly method that can be given either to individual PBL teams or to the cohort as a whole. Use of technology such as computerised statistical packages and optical scanning equipment produces results in a short time, ready for perusal and action if required. Care is required in the selection and wording of items to be evaluated. Rating scales can be incorporated either in the form of numerical values or quality statements (very satisfactory to very unsatisfactory for example). The number of items to be evaluated and the timing of issue of the questionnaire require consideration. Evaluative questionnaires are often administered at the end of modules or programmes. Students may become bored with questionnaires, especially if there are many items. Administering several multi-item questionnaires at one point in the programme can lead students to 'switch off' and fail to give full consideration to every item.

Where detail is required, a qualitative approach to evaluation is preferable. These include observational methods such as facilitator notes and video or audio-taping. As indicated above, the introduction of an outside person into an established team will alter the dynamics of the team, even if the person does not participate in the PBL process but acts only as a observer. One way of overcoming this may be to video film the session. It can be argued that the presence of a video camera is just as intrusive as another person. However once the camera is set up, team members become used to it and forget its presence, especially if video taping is a frequent occurrence. The videotape can be viewed by the team and evaluation of performance made by self, peers and facilitator. Facilitator performance can also be evaluated from the video. Students can be involved in this process. Alternatively, the tape can be used for self-evaluation. Viewing of the tape by another facilitator can be used to provide peer review for the facilitator and can give an outsider perspective on the workings of the team. Audio-taping can be used in a similar way. In both strategies students can take control of the taping equipment and can be involved in deciding which PBL seminars should be taped. It is useful for a complete 'set' of PBL sessions (introduction, reviews and feedback) to be taped in order to provide a comprehensive picture of the workings of the team. It is not unusual for a PBL team to perform better in one type of session. Having the whole set of seminars will highlight this and allow discussion around improvement of the less favoured sessions. Evaluation can be undertaken by use of focus groups (Bloor *et al.*, 2001). This technique requires the participation of students in the focus group. Selection of students may be random – students may be asked to select one or two members from each PBL team or volunteers may be sought. All of the selection methods have disadvantages. Students who volunteer may have non-representative views on PBL; students elected by PBL teams may not be interested and random selection may not cover all student perspectives. As focus groups are additional to the work required by the programme, attendance may be problematic. Focus groups operate by giving members two or three questions on topics of concern and asking for discussion. In some respects, this is similar to the introductory PBL seminars, so should not be threatening for students. The discussion is taped and notes are made by the person running the discussion. Review of the tape transcripts together with the notes provides detailed information about the topics raised. This information can be used to inform further programme developments.

The role of the facilitator in evaluation

Facilitation is a combination of modelling the desired learning behaviours and scaffolding support for students. As the team becomes more expert in utilising the PBL process, facilitator intervention decreases and the supporting scaffold is gradually withdrawn. Evaluating one's own performance is an aspect that students often find difficult initially. It is therefore one of the desired behaviours to be modelled as part of the development of critical thinking skills. Facilitators need to model behaviour on giving and receiving criticism in a positive, constructive and non-threatening manner. Evaluative comments should be made about behaviour or material and should not be personally addressed. They should also indicate that they reflect the speaker's perspective. Some suggestions for improving behaviour could also be included in facilitative comments. Using evaluative techniques requires considerable courage, understanding and mutual respect. It is important that qualitative evaluation is based on what has actually taken place rather than the evaluator's interpretation of what has happened.

The first stage in formative evaluation can be linked to reflection. As discussed above, students should develop skills in judging the quality of their own work. This can be initiated by asking students to consider the material brought to the feedback session and its relationship to the learning outcomes set for the seminar by the students. As the material is distant from the student, it is relatively comfortable to reflect on. When students are familiar with this process they can then be encouraged to reflect on their contribution to the team in terms of assisting the team to move forward in addition to finding material to support arguments. Students need not be asked to share their reflections at first. Facilitators can use modelling behaviours to encourage students in their reflection by offering an example of their own behaviour such as 'I felt that I gave you too much direction at the start of that last trigger'. Students may find reflection difficult to begin with and tend to describe what they did without considering the effect of their action. If students are to progress to sharing their reflections with other members of the team and offering evaluation to each other, safety and trust are essential. Confidentiality within the team is usually set as a ground rule (see Chapters 2 and 4). Wolff (1998) suggests that behaviour rather than personal characteristics should be the focus as behaviours can be more readily altered than personality. Facilitators need to ensure that evaluation is assistive and does not become destructive, for example reminding the team that members should each be allowed to have a say rather than telling one member that he is overbearing. Inferences should be clearly identified as such – 'it seemed to me that ...' rather than as statements of fact. Students then have a chance to respond to a misinterpretation rather than wondering why that angle has been taken.

Care should be taken with voice tone and non-verbal cues especially during evaluation. The words themselves may be suitable but the meaning can be altered by voice cadence and facial expression.

Activity 8.4
What do you think the following sentence means?
You did that very well
Try to change the meaning of the sentence by changing your tone of voice, the emphasis on words or your facial expression and ask a colleague what they think that sentence means.

> **Commentary 8.4**
> On first reading you probably gave each word equal emphasis, making the sentence sound like positive evaluation. If you put different stress on each word, then the meaning is altered.
>
> For example
> *You* did that very well = the others did it badly
> You did *that* very well = but you do other things less well
> You did that *very* well = your usual performance is good, but this was even better
> You did that very well? = I don't think you did, do you think you did well?

Even if the facilitator does not speak, students are often cue conscious and will interpret (or misinterpret) non-verbal communication such as facial expression, gestures or body position. Trying not to give non-verbal cues is difficult and can be interpreted as disinterest by the students. Non-verbal cues, such as nodding or smiling, can be used positively to encourage students to expand on a fruitful theme or to draw students into the discussion without interrupting the flow of talk.

The above section relates to verbal, face-to-face evaluation, usually incorporated into the feedback seminar. It is possible to construct questionnaires to seek and provide information on team processes. Questions that are used by the student as self-assessment (such as the questions in figure 8.1), can be re-phrased to be used by facilitators to evaluate students' performance in PBL. A rating scale can be added if a more formal evaluation is desired. Such scales can be simple or complex. Simple scales require the rater to indicate whether or not the student has exhibited a particular behaviour during the seminar, for example:

Did the student contribute to the discussion?   yes/no
Had the student prepared material for the
  PBL session?   yes/no

Scales can be more complex and require the rater to quantify, often on a Likert-type scale, for example:

How appropriate were the student's contributions?
Very appropriate, appropriate, not very appropriate, inappropriate.
The student included other students in the discussion.
Always, sometimes, never.

Completion of such scales is a complex activity, requiring the facilitator, not only to follow the argument presented by each individual student during the seminar, but to rate objectively each of the students and their interactions.

Acting on findings

Part of the planning for evaluating PBL is the decision about who should receive the evaluation and the use to which the findings will be put. Evaluation of seminar performance may not be recorded, especially if undertaken orally. Students may make notes of the evaluation for personal use. Facilitators may also record the main points of the evaluation and use these in the future to highlight any improvement or regression of performance. However, the evaluation remains confidential to the facilitator and the team. If evaluation is undertaken on a more formal basis, the findings from all PBL teams in a cohort may be combined and used to form part of, for example, a modular or annual report. Combining of evaluation in this method helps to identify difficulties common to all teams. Reports on the wider issues of the PBL curriculum should be provided for facilitators, students and also those individuals within an institution who have responsibilities for timetabling and resourcing to inform discussion on further developments.

Conclusion

Evaluation in PBL relates to the PBL process and also the wider issues associated with the organisation of a problem-based curriculum. Time for evaluation of the PBL process should be timetabled in advance. Evaluation should consider student and facilitator performance and be undertaken in a format that will provide sufficiently detailed information. Methods for in-seminar performance include use of facilitator notes (non-)participant observation, pre-prepared rating scales, audio-or video taping, focus teams and questionnaires. Wider curricular issues can be evaluated by questionnaires, focus teams and by combination of in-seminar evaluations. PBL is a resource intensive strategy, which requires sound organisation, good facilitation and adequate resources if students are to achieve the benefits. Student attrition is a major concern for schools and departments of nursing. Evaluation of programmes is essential to identify good practice and to establish where improvements are needed.

References

Bloor, M, Frankland, J, Thomas, M and Robson, K (2001) Focus Groups in Social Research, London: Sage.

de Grave, W, Dolmans, D H J M and van der Vleuten, C P M (1998) Tutor intervention profile: reliability and validity, *Medical Education*, **32**: 262–8.

Dolmans, D H J M, Wolfhagen, I A P and Snellen-Balendong, H A M (1994) Improving the effectiveness of tutors in problem-based learning, *Medical Teacher*, **16**(4): 369–77.

Robinson, A (1995) Transformative 'cultural shifts' in nursing: participatory action research and the 'project of possibility', *Nursing Inquiry*, **2**: 65–74.

Schön, D (1987) *Educating the Reflective Practitioner*, London: Jossey-Bass.

Schwartz, P, Mennin, S and Webb, G (eds) (2001) *Problem-based Learning. Case Studies, Experience and Practice*, London: Kogan Page.

Wilkie, K (2002) *Actions, Attitudes and Attributes: Developing skills for facilitation in problem-based learning*, Unpublished Thesis, University of Coventry.

Wolff, A C (1998) *The Role of the Tutor in Context-based Learning. An Orientation Guide for Nursing Faculty*, Alberta: University of Alberta.

Index